BOB LIPTON & LISA MACALLEN PHD

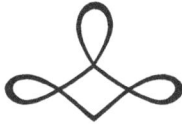

STOP OVERTHINKING:

REBALANCE YOURSELF. A DETAILED GUIDE
ON HOW TO BREAK NEGATIVE HABITS AND
MASTER YOUR EMOTIONS. STOP WORRYING
CYCLES, INCREASE YOUR CONFIDENCE AND
LEARN HOW TO DECLUTTER YOUR MIND.

Table Of Contents

Introduction

These days, the stress in life has increased so much that people have started thinking that peace is the goal of life, it isn't. Peace is the way of life and leading a meaningful and constructive life should be the goal. Even the animals and birds that do not have the same cognitive abilities as ours lead a peaceful life. There is no reason for this life not to be peaceful or be chaotic until some external force is applied.

Now it is time to go on and make your life happier. This tip is to not hold on to the mistakes and events that have happened in the past. It is crucial always to be mindful that the past is already done and you are not able to do anything about what you did in the past. This can be a challenging thing for many people to deal with. They may remember something that they said or did, or maybe something that someone else said or did in the past and want to hold on to it for years to come. This isn't worth it if it is not making you happy at all. Instead, it is making you feel depressed.

Does it make you feel good to sit there and concentrate all that energy on being negative about the whole situation? Do you get anything accomplished by doing this or do you just feel mad, jealous, and a little drained? Rather than letting these negative emotions take control of your life and make you feel unhappy; you need to learn how to turn them around and feel true happiness. For example, you can sit there and think about how great of a job they have been doing in their new position, making it a lot easier for you to get your work done, and it must have been all that hard work in the presentation for the new client that got them the promotion over you.

It is also possible to get into a fight with your family and friends over something that does not matter all that much to either of you, just neither wanted to lose. How many friends have you lost from the past just because they did not continue to hold the same kinds of values or thoughts that you did? Maybe it goes back to high school and you and your best friend got in a fight over a boy that you both liked. Or perhaps you have not talked to your mother for a few months because she disapproved of a decision you were trying to make.

How do you feel about these situations all this time later? Hopefully in the case of fighting over a boy in high school with your friend, you have gotten over it and perhaps are even talking to the friend again. But with some of the other arguments that you have had, does it make you feel that great not to see or speak to the ones that you love. Most likely the answer is no.

To be completely happy in your life, you need to learn to let the things that are harming you in your life go. It does not matter who was right and who was wrong in the whole scenario. If something is not working out, you and the other person need to take the time to figure out what that something is, work on fixing it, and then put the whole situation in the past rather than holding on to it for years to come. Dwelling on the past is a surefire way to make everyone feel bad and it is not healthy in the least. You should be concentrating all of your efforts on the bright future that is before you rather than on the dark things and mistakes that have made up your past. Yes, mistakes are what shape you into the person who you are today, but that does not mean that they are bringing you any happiness by holding on to them.

CHAPTER 1:

Awareness is the Beginning of Change

The Importance of Acknowledging Your Overthinking Issue

While you overthink, in preference to acting and doing things, you're over thinking. While you examine, comment and repeat the same thoughts over and again, instead of performing, you're over thinking.

This addiction obstructs you from taking action. It consumes your strength, disables your ability to make choices, and places you on a loop of wondering and thinking over and once more. This is a sort of thinking that wastes some time and energy and prevents you from appearing, doing new matters and making progress in your life.

It's like tying yourself to a rope that is related to a pole and moving into circles time and again. When you don't over think, you emerge as greener, more nonviolent and extra satisfied.

Your issues should be dealt with. Running from it will not solve anything. The very first step is realizing that you have an issue in solving it.

You just can't stop thinking about an event, someone, something that passed off in the beyond, or on a hassle. Rather than searching out an answer, taking initiative and being lively, you just hold questioning and can't get it out of your thoughts.

At instances, while something terrible takes place, you consider the worst scenarios, with thoughts like "what if?" or "why?" You slip now after which into terrible questioning styles.

You worry approximately past mistakes or present-day problems and troubles, and the way they might result in bad results. You inflate every phrase, notion, and event beyond truly and reasonable proportions, studying into its things that aren't certainly there.

Be Honest with Yourself

If you do no longer have a time-restrict for while you need to make a choice and take action then you may just preserve turning your thoughts approximately think about them from all angles to your thoughts for a very long term.

So, discover ways to grow to be better at making decisions and to spring into movement using putting time limits for each day existence. Regardless of if it's a small or more extensive selection.

Because how you begin your day tends to set the tone in your day regularly.

Honesty is a very essential tool if you want your life to go smooth sailing. It doesn't only mean that you have to be honest. In most cases, it means that you have to be realistic enough to know where you're coming from. The ones matter which can look poor have taught them loads and have been priceless to help them to grow.

So, prevent seeking to manipulate the whole thing. Trying to do so truly doesn't work because nobody can see all the feasible situations in advance.

This is of directionless difficult stated than executed. So, do it in small steps if you want.

And not just human beings and corporations near you in actual lifestyles. But additionally, what you examine, pay attention to and watch. The blogs, books, boards, films, podcasts and track in your existence.

To reflect on consideration on if there are any resources to your life – nearby or similarly away – that encourages and tends to create extra over thinking to your thoughts. And think about what humans or assets that has the opposite impact on you.

Locate ways to spend extra of sometime and interest with the human beings and input which have an advantageous effect on your questioning and much less on the impact that tends to bolster your over thinking dependency.

Release Fears to Explore the Unknown

Fear has to be set free! Maintaining terror is acknowledging the harmful possibilities which fear depicts.

When addressing it face-on you will unleash anxiety and eradicate it and then just go through with it. Only without the harmful effects that anxiety reflects by diminishing your future away and strengthening that fear within, you can't even hold into it.

The further power we create in becoming solid, stable and transparent, so more opportunities we might manage to push through challenges, challenges and results we'd been afraid of. Teach yourselves alike, teaching oneself is a subconscious-based practice which demonstrates the brain what to do to deal with the possibilities which accompany the worries successfully. Many times than otherwise, learning lets people proceed to point one, to enable people to discharge their fears and therefore permitting it to dismiss many other concerns explicitly only with a little bit knowledge.

If you've had a deep fear of doing something, now you can perform outwardly to educate you methods to respond with or explore some these worries more cleanly. Throughout this be careful with oneself. For just a cause, we have had some concerns, but still look at the fears initially and see if that's anything that helps people escape a major issue ahead of you. Only redesign those acts appropriately. Frequently anxiety is a tale that you keep it onto, and so we can change the situation to expel fear.

Signs That You Are Overthinking

Do you discover it hard to close off your mind at any given moment? Do you sense exhausted and nerve-racking due to your thoughts? In that case, you're possibly a persistent over thinker. Sadly, over thinking has emerged as a global epidemic, as we live in complicated instances that require a lot of brainpower from us. Responsibilities, budget, emotional trauma, and other problems depart our minds in a state of overdrive. Through vast studies, psychology professors discovered that young and middle elderly adults mainly engage in over thinking, with 73% of 25-35 12 months-olds diagnosed as over thinkers. No longer extraordinarily, extra ladies (fifty-seven %) than guys (43%) identify as over thinkers.

So, when you have trouble detaching from your thoughts and experience consistently confused using them, we have a few guidelines under to help you forestall over thinking, and common signs that your mind has overtaken you.

Normal Insomnia

Over thinkers recognize the problem of falling asleep all too nicely. Insomnia takes a keep on you because you couldn't seem to shut off your mind, and the thoughts slowly paralyze you. Your thoughts races and also you sense too stressed to sleep; all the worries from the day hold flooding your mind, and you may break out from this mental prison. If this sounds to you, seek to do fun activities earlier than bed, like mindfulness, exercise, painting, and drawing, reporting, reading, or perhaps speaking to a loved one. Do something that keeps off your mind from moving to something else that enables your imagination and feelings to return to the ground.

Dwelling in Worry

In case you stay in fear of destiny, then you simply are trapped in your thoughts. Fear reasons over thinkers to show drugs or alcohol on the way to drown their terrible mind.

Other guidelines could be to allow a "window" for the over thinking. Allot 15 to 30 minutes in keeping with day to get out all of your concerns, whether thru writing or speak to a person. This manner, you can carry on with your day and depart the worries in the dust.

Overanalyzing the Entirety

Over thinkers have one significant hassle: they have got a want to govern the whole lot? They want to devise out the future, however, because they cannot expect it, this reasons them excellent tension. They don't like dealing with whatever they can't manipulate. They have a prime worry of the unknown, which causes them to take a seat and mull over all of the options as opposed to taking movement.

When you locate yourself over thinking, attempt to carry yourself again to the existing second via deep breaths and thinking about something that relaxes you. Attempt to think about how these thoughts will serve you inside the gift second, and this alone should remove them, as you'll discover that they do not anything for you but motive notable strain.

Fear of Failure

Over thinkers also have a constant choice for perfection in the entirety they do. They cannot take delivery of failure, and do the whole thing of their energy to keep away from it. Ironically, this typically includes doing not anything. Keep in mind, the over-thinker is paralyzed by fear, so instead of facing defeat, instead they would rather not be in a position to lose.

If that sounds like you, note you're so much more than just the faults and screw-ups. However, note that you have to commit specific errors to get everywhere in life. These will allow you in your evolution to develop, research, and attain new heights.

Continuously Second-Guessing Your Self

Due to their preference for perfection, over thinkers continually analyze, reanalyze, and triple examine any scenario. They don't want to make the wrong choice, so that they take an entirely long time to make any preference, due to the fact they don't trust themselves. They're out of contact with their intuition, so each decision comes from the mind, and this isn't continually a great aspect. If the brain is so foggy and bogged down that you may make a precise selection, then you definitely an over thinker.

Lack of Ability to Stay Inside the Present Moment

If you can't even live inside the gift moment and enjoy life as it comes, then you are a sufferer of over thinking. Wondering an excessive amount of causes you to lose awareness of the sector around you, and turn out to be trapped in your mind. Becoming bogged down with mind eliminates you from the now, and might disrupt your relationships with others.

Don't forget to open your mind and heart to the world around you, and no longer get so wrapped up in bad thinking. Handiest allow thoughts into your brain that serve your well-being and try and ignore the ones that best convey you down. Lifestyles gives so much beauty and the possibility for extraordinary stories. Still, you can handiest admire this in case you discover ways to track from your mind and into your coronary heart instead.

The Psychology behind Chronic Overthinking

Because everybody sometimes overthinks some very issues, chronic excessive-thinkers waste much of their waking moments obsessing; and that clamps down on themselves. Instead of pressure, they confuse it with stress. 'Should haves' and 'what ifs' govern their thoughts, as if an unseen jury is sitting on their lives in judgment. And they're also agonizing on what to say online as they're highly worried about how others view their comments as well as new features.

Additionally, relationships with others help to silence one's weak thoughts. While we take note of others, we provide ourselves damage and consequently put the focal point on a person else. Learn to live in reality, pay attention to others, bond with them, and ask them questions about their lives. We can prevent this chronic over thinking problem together via forming communities once more and studying to aid and hook up with each other.

CHAPTER 2:

The Power of Your Thoughts

How Your Thoughts Control Your Outcome and How it Will Reflect Your Reality

Y ou, your resilience, and your capacity for growth are much more reliable than your anxious thoughts—although it probably doesn't feel like that most of the time. For the troubled mind, a flood of worry can rise in a matter of minutes, sweeping you away to a place where what began as a passing thought becomes in your head an absolute truth. When you look closely at your feelings you might well draw yourself leaping to extreme measures and assumptions.

Imagine you get a ticket for a minor fender bender and then you have the thought, "What if they sue me?" Anxiety quickly evolves that thought into, "They are going to sue me!" Or say you get some negative feedback at work and have the thought, "My boss sees problems with my work." Anxiety steps in, and the thought becomes, "I'm going to get fired." Or you realize your mom hasn't returned your phone calls and you wonder why. Anxiety turns wondering into, "She must have had an accident." Or you realize your partner hasn't returned a text all day and you worry, "My partner doesn't care about me anymore," quickly followed by, "He's leaving me!" A physical sensation can also initiate this pattern of taking one small, worrisome thought to an extreme: "My heart is beating fast . . . I must be having a heart attack!" There are all sorts of frightening, unlikely places your anxious thoughts will take you—but only if you let them! Believe it or not, you can intervene and slow this process down.

Imagining catastrophes and worst-case scenarios is emotionally draining and keeps us from being fully present in the here and now. But we can learn to sort our thoughts so that things like over-the-top speculations and black-and-white thinking are moved to the "discard" pile, at least until you have solid evidence that those thoughts are realistic. Start sorting helpful from unhelpful thoughts by taking a little time (even if only a few moments) to slow down and become aware of what you're thinking before you react.

Expectations: What They are and Where they Come From

When we experience normal anxiety, we focus on the immediate concerns and challenges that no one is immune to, e.g., "Thanksgiving with the family is going to be hard to get through this year." The highly anxious mind compounds these difficulties by extending them out across time and over a variety of situations: "Every time I'm with my family, I get stressed out." Even worse, the anxious mind convinces us that we won't be able to cope with the thing we dread: "I can't go to any more family functions, it's too upsetting." We tend to have different expectations to the scenarios we play in our head. As a result, we spin our wheels trying to prevent feared situations, emotions, and/or interactions by avoiding people and events that don't pose a real threat. Of course, in reality, there's only so much control we have throughout events, and so all this anxious energy results in us feeling at the mercy of life, powerless, and desperate to find relief.

Why We Imagine Things and Play out Scenario's in our Mind

When we expect, we develop conclusions about ourselves, our emotions, and what we can and can't do based on a single experience. For instance, Carmen found out she didn't get her desired work promotion and concludes: "I'll never get promoted." Nolan had a couple of unfulfilling dates and concludes: "I'll never meet the right one."

Imagining things causes you to seal the deal on your fate. In your mind, you render your future chances of success or getting what you want at zero. And perhaps most importantly, imagining means an end to trying.

Sometimes, we tend to underestimate our ability to cope if what we fear happens. We tell ourselves we can't possibly manage the frightening situation our mind is generating: "No way, I wouldn't even know what to do," "I won't be able to deal with that," "That would kill me," "I'd go crazy." In the face of a possible adversity, we imagine ourselves melting into a puddle of anxious fear. This reinforces the superstitious notion that worry itself will keep us safe: "If I worry enough, I'll be okay," "If I obsess over this project, I'll work harder," "If I keep myself upset and on edge about this, I'll be better prepared when it happens."

This pattern can be broken. You're capable of managing far more than you imagine. Just because you don't want to deal with something, or it may be hard to deal with, doesn't mean you can't be effective. You have already managed quite a bit in your life. You just do it; you push through to the other side.

When Our Expectations Do Not Occur How It Makes Us Feel

When we're caught up in anxious thinking, our thoughts feel entirely real and accurate and so they keep us keyed up. In truth, the anxious mind isn't so good at differentiating the real from the unreal. In this virtual world, we feel as anxious and frightened as we would if our fear was based on something happening. However, in reality, nothing terrible is going on and there may be little, if any, chance our feared scenarios will ever happen.

There are several biases we're all prone to that intensify anxiety. Familiarizing yourself with these "errors in thinking" will help you catch exaggerated or inaccurate thought patterns. Below are some of the known types:

All-or-nothing thinking: Things are all good or all bad; you are perfect or a failure.

Overgeneralizing: If something negative happens in one situation it means it will happen in all future, similar situations.

Catastrophizing: You look to the future with sweeping negativity and forecast disaster instead of more realistic possibilities.

Labeling: Applying a fixed, global label on yourself or others without including any context. ("I'm a loser," "I'm bad," "I'm inadequate," "I'm a burden.")

"Should"-ing and "must"-ing: You have rigid expectations for how you should or must act, and when these unreasonable expectations aren't met, you forecast horrendous consequences.

Each time you successfully identify an error in thinking, your anxiety will decrease because you're able to see the situation at hand more realistically, or at least entertain other possibilities.

Releasing Expectations: How to Live More Freely

When we are caught in anxiety quicksand, each and every worrisome thought may seem acute and reasonable. Stress hormones are released, anxiety builds, and it becomes difficult to distinguish the probable from the possible. Instead of repeating the same concerns over and over in your head, write out the following for each of your uneasy expectations:

- What is the worst possible scenario that I'm afraid of happening regarding this thought?
- What is the best possible scenario that I wish could happen regarding this thought?
- What is a realistic scenario that will likely happen regarding this thought?

You can be at peace. Slow down and train your mind to steer away from far-reaching catastrophe and toward thoughts that represent the realistic, and most likely, outcomes.

Perhaps you're recognizing some of your anxious thinking represents expectation. Nonetheless, you still can't get the fear or thought out of your mind. Start challenging those expectations. When you hit a setback, ask yourself the following questions—and write your responses down, if you can.

1. Can you think of a time in the past when your conclusion has not been true?

2. Can you imagine a time or instance in the future when your conclusion may not be true?

3. How probable, from 0 to 100 percent, do you feel it is that the fear you're thinking about is going actually to happen?

4. What do you gain by believing this thought? For example, do you think it keeps you safe in some way?

5. What consequences may come from believing this thought? For example, will you give up trying to get what you desire, allowing a self-fulfilling prophecy to result?

How to Change your Perspective in Life

1. Think through one of your more upsetting thoughts or worst-case scenarios. In your mind's eye, play out the details of what you fear as if it is really happening. Imagine where you are, whom you are interacting with, or what news you're getting.

2. Now imagine your worst-case blocks, setbacks, or embarrassments, but visualize yourself effectively coping with what you're feeling or the other feared obstacles.

3. Instead of freaking out, giving up, or becoming painfully uncomfortable with anxiety or fear, you stick with the situation. People are being motivated to figure out a way to deal with your biggest fear effectively.

4. Imagine you use a strategy (take a few deep breaths, use internal supportive language, remind yourself of your larger goals) and it works. You show yourself that you can cope. You find a way through the circumstances and emerge in a more comfortable and thoughtful place.

5. Always have gratitude. This is the last key in order for your life to sail smoothly. Being grateful not only affects your mood but also the

mood of the people around you. If you always practice this strategy, you will always have a positive outlook in life.

Being Responsible for Your Life, Thoughts and Actions

It is our direct responsibility to take good care of our thoughts. These thoughts will always reflect on out actions. May it be a good or a bad thought, it will come out on its own no matter how we try to hide it. As we all know, we will be judged based on our actions. There's plenty of moments in our existence in which we regret something that we did because it somehow reflected on who we are. Thus, we should always be careful in whatever we say and do. We only have one life. We should see to it that we live it morally and ethically good for us to avoid regrets later in life.

The Benefits of Allowing Yourself a Different Perspective

The situation is not at fault. It's your perspective that always matters.

Far too often we find "progress" or "doing just what we enjoy" as that of a goal. It's a place we need to get to. What some of us fail to understand is that all of these concepts are something of a process solution, not really the conclusion of the journey.

As you walk that journey you are "productive," continually improving, always rising. You 'do what you value' if you see each time as something of a chance. Explore what this opportunity can do to your life.

Where many Kids and adolescents tend to be irritated, they view it all as inevitable. They think, "I'm trapped now," they look towards their basement work as that of the bottom, there seems to be nowhere to go and they think as if they're not going to hit the "win" intended outcome.

Yet no matter where it is located, or what you do, things have to be experienced. And till you can explore such teachings then follow your personal path; you just cannot truly achieve the "good" condition of sensation.

CHAPTER 3:

Basic Emotional Needs

What Are Our Basic Emotional Needs?

Sometimes, emotions arise for no apparent reason. Sometimes, it is due to some internal or external factors. The emotional state of a person can be very dynamic, especially if the person has not learned how to control his or her feelings.

If you perceive the same occasion positively, you will appear more relaxed. You will also feel some excitement as the day of the occasion approaches. These are two different kinds of emotions arising from the same occurrence. That means that how you view life and the events in it determines how your emotions behave.

Each emotion always comprises of two components – a physical component and a mental component. These two also affect a person's mood and feelings differently. The mental part of emotions is characterized by:

- The ability to differentiate and choose between pain and pleasure
- The tendency to engage inactivity
- Memory thought, and perception of an individual. These three aspects define the social, mental, and material interests of human beings
- Ability to differentiate between muscular and organic sensations

- The bodily component of emotions, on the other hand, determines:
- Any changes in the body's internal organs as a result of emotional changes
- Movement of body muscles

The mental component is what comprises an emotional experience while the bodily part is what is known as emotional expression. Basically, emotion is often triggered by the imagination, thought, or perception of a particular circumstance. It is not triggered by a single thing or event but a collection of mental activities.

External occurrences cause different kinds of emotions. For instance, seeing a leopard always triggers fear of getting harmed or losing a life. However, seeing the same leopard in a cage will not trigger the emotion of fear.

Every emotion is a response to a situation. It can be pleasant or painful, depending on your perception of the situation.

Some Conditions That Affect Our Emotional Needs

The way you perceive others also determines how you interact with them. For instance, when you have a negative perception towards others, you may find that the responses you give them are somewhat hostile even if the question asked was a simple one. If you have a positive perception towards others, your engagement with them will be a fulfilling one, and you will leave them happy. It is, therefore, vital that you control your perception to ensure that you appear emotionally intelligent.

Your mental health can also affect your emotions. Stress and the lack of stress always manifest physically as well as emotionally. Physical manifestations of stress may include muscle aches and general body pain. Emotional signs are things like anger, sadness, and anxiety. Your stress levels significantly affect your mood. It is therefore crucial that you learn how to manage your stress by identifying the source of the stress and dealing with it appropriately.

Lack of sleep impacts your general mood during the day. It is always enjoyed staying up late, especially when doing something that is fun. However, doing this continuously can interfere with the functional ability of your body. You may start feeling moody all the time, and this may result in severe health conditions like stroke and heart problems. To relieve yourself from such occurrences, always ensure that you get enough sleep. The recommended hours of sleep for every individual is between seven and nine hours. If you are an early riser, it is essential that you sleep early enough.

Hormones can also cause emotions to fluctuate significantly. For example, women whose bodies have low levels of estrogen hormone may notice drastic changes in their emotions. Testosterone hormone levels may also cause a mood problem in men. Tests can be carried out to determine if hormones are responsible for the mood changes experienced by a person.

Some foods may be responsible for mood fluctuations as well. For instance, chocolate causes a trigger in sugar levels and endorphins. This results in a feeling of pleasantness and excitement.

Your surrounding dramatically determines the kind of emotions you generate. A home or place that is adorned with bright, shiny colors will always make you happy and at ease. The surrounding alone will improve your mood significantly. However, places like call centers or chat rooms with dull walls, and nothing colorful in place will always create a gloomy environment. There is nothing exciting about such situations. This explains why most workplaces do not get too many decorations.

Workplaces are not placing of excitement but places of serious business. However, your overall mood always affects how you respond to certain situations. For instance, if you are in a gloomy environment and a challenging issue arises, your response may not be quite good, especially if you have had quite a long day. If you have been confined in such an environment for long hours, you may feel frustrated by the new issue that has arisen and may end up getting angry at everyone.

Most interior designers understand the place of colors in determining the mood in the room. For instance, most people use white and gray in the workroom, yet research shows that individuals who work in rooms painted in these colors tend to become less active and productive.

One example of individuals who get overwhelmed with the work environment is call center representatives. They are always faced with an expectation that some cannot meet. Customers always expect them to remain confident and joyful at all times, regardless of how their day has been. However, this sometimes becomes impossible, and their emotions may run beyond control.

Besides colors, the lighting of an environment may also trigger negative or positive emotions. For instance, blue lights often promote a sense of creativity in the workplace and create a calm environment in the home. Studies show that being exposed to blue lighting improves performance significantly. Natural light also plays a significant role in the home or work environment. It causes people to relax more, giving them better control of their emotions.

Ways to Address and Understand Our Emotional Needs

There are certain times in our lives when we feel dissatisfied or frustrated about something. There are even times when we don't know the reason why we are feeling sad. Each one of us has their own emotional needs to be satisfied. Sometimes, we feel like we are not safe in a particular place and that causes triggers to our mental health. We then overthink and remember a moment in the past where we felt afraid and unsecured in a place.

If we do not try to overcome these thoughts, it will haunt us. It will then link back to our childhood wounds that we hoped to be forgotten forever. That is why it is essential that we address and understand our emotional needs.

How Our Emotional Needs Affect Our Thoughts

There are emotions that cause people to react in a certain way, and this affects how a person thinks. This is always helpful when danger is involved. Sometimes, things happen, and there is no time to think before acting, but there are some emotions that trigger a lot of thinking. For example, if you encounter a person that is undergoing a challenge, the feeling of sympathy or sorrow may cause you to start thinking about how you will assist the person.

Negative emotions mostly lead to negative thoughts, while positive emotions often lead to positive thoughts. That is why it is essential that you change your way of thinking. For example, if you sit an exam and fail it, you may start thinking that you will never pass the exam, and this assumption may cause you to stop working hard. When this happens, you should analyze the situation to understand better why you failed in the first place. This will help you to improve on the areas that need development so that you can perform better next time.

Most emotions often show in the person's face or actions. A good example is when you are angry. You will either raise your voice at others or make somebody's movements that suggest your agitation. The anger may also show on your face as frowns or clenched teeth. Some of these actions are predictable, while others occur without expectation.

Actions always indicate an expression of feelings. That is why it is not advisable to suppress your feelings, even if they are negative. Trying to suppress your emotions can cause mental and physical problems.

When it comes to behavior, emotions also affect the way a person makes decisions. Negative emotions always trigger negative decisions since they make people feel like they have minimal options available. When you are excited, you are still bound to make unrealistic decisions that are regrettable. That is why it's advisable that you do not make decisions when highly agitated or highly excited.

As for the workplace, emotions can impact the motivation, personality, and temperament of a person.

They cloud a person's sense of perception and judgment. Emotions also play a significant role in determining how you react to the stimuli that occur in your environment. When you are exposed to negative emotions for a long time, you may develop some sicknesses such as ulcers and heart problems. This also applies to stressful environments at work and at home. Generally having a bad mood always reduces the performance of individuals since this makes employees make poor decisions that may affect the company's overall performance.

On the other hand, a positive wave of emotions boosts problem-solving and creativity skills of employees. As earlier stated, emotions are caused by a chemical balance in the brain. This chemical balance always determines an individual's mood and energy level. It also enhances or diminishes one's thinking and judgment capabilities. Individuals must, therefore, seek to identify how their emotional state affects their behavior as a way of improving how they interact with others and respond to situations. Positive emotions always lead to satisfaction; therefore, it is still essential to ensure that your emotions are adequately balanced.

How Emotions Can Link Back to Childhood Wounds

Although painful incidents may occur to anybody, we are far more prone to be deeply affected by such an event if you are already experiencing intense pressure, has experienced a set of defeats lately, or have been previously emotionally scarred — especially if the previous trauma has happened during childhood.

Trauma to childhood may arise from something that interferes with a kid's feeling of security, such as:

- A fragile or dangerous condition
- Parental separation
- Serious disease
- Disruptive clinical interventions
- Sexual, emotional or physical violence
- Domestic abuse

Suffering childhood abuse could indeed lead to severe and prolonged impacts. Once trauma to the childhood is not addressed, a feeling of anxiety as well as desperation passes to adult years, laying the groundwork for even more trauma. But also though the trauma occurred several years earlier, you will heal the agony, begin to accept and re-connect with everyone, and over time recover the deep emotions.

CHAPTER 4:

Why Life is Difficult When We Overthink

U ltimately, there are many complications which can arise when you suffer from an overly active mind—you can suffer from many different degrees of stress, panic or anxiety attacks, you may lash out at others, or even worse physical complications when you only keep piling on more and more stress. Although it can be challenging to set aside time for yourself so that you can alleviate all this stress, it's endlessly essential to understand precisely what can happen to you if you don't keep yourself in check mentally—being aware of the way you can devolve emotionally is an excellent way to make sure you understand the gravity of your mental health, and you take as best care of yourself as possible.

Of course, the first and most obvious reason that you should try to keep yourself away from indulging in overactive thinking is stress. Stress can come in many forms, and it can be incredibly challenging to get rid of in large amounts.

Of course, there is also an unhealthy kind of stress. This happens when we let healthy stress build and build over a long period of time without doing anything to vent it or allow it to dissipate over time naturally. If we have a project, we keep putting off, the healthy stress to do work becomes unhealthy stress out of fear of failure or fear of punishment if you were to keep putting the work off. There's only one kind of stress, but whether or not it ends up being healthy or unhealthy tends to rely solely on the person experiencing the stress and how they deal with the stress on their own. Someone who is generally social and makes plans with their friends might feel the healthy stress to make the get-together a success and catch up. Someone who isn't as social or is less used to going out with other people might feel more unhealthy stress due to anxiety over the meetup. This is due to a lot of different factors—some people are just naturally less accustomed to stress and never learned how to deal with it properly, and some people are also born less able to handle stress. While part of this trait is nature, and part is nurture, the reason that healthy stress becomes unhealthy stress can also depend on the specific situation. If someone is feeling a lot of stress, either necessarily healthy or unhealthy, they have a few choices as to how they can deal with that stress. They can either do what they're stressing out over, or relieve stress naturally through facing the point of their stress, or they can actively ignore their potentially healthy stress and let it build up into more troubling, unhealthy strain on the mind and body. When this happens, the individual is more prone to anxiety or panic attacks from that intense stress. They're more likely to have a breakdown over that stress because they haven't had the opportunity to vent it, and other complications are much more likely to arise over the failure to deal with that stress properly. In this position, the person feeling the stress has probably put off their responsibilities and has, in turn, had to deal with the extra stress of that decision. The decisions which people make every day also tend to majorly impact the kind of stress they'll have, the type of day they will have based on the kind of stress and level of that stress, and the type of stress they're more likely to lead if they keep making the kinds of decisions they make presently as it pertains to whether they have healthy stress, which they deal with properly and can vent if need be, or unhealthy stress which plagues them for a long time after when someone with healthy stress may have vented their stresses. The unhealthy choices made by busy people directly impacts the life they will lead.

Anxiety can come from many different things—anxiety can develop during childhood or from behaviors we pick up when we're young, much like stress. If we live our childhood with our parents or environment placing a lot of unhealthy pressure on us about performance, tests, or doing well in school, we will likely become more afraid of taking tests and afraid of presenting our achievements to others—we fear the failure that may come with that trust we have in others. When a certain pressure is heavily placed on us in childhood, it tends to follow us up through our high school years through college, and even into our adult lives. Though perhaps we "should be" focusing on doing the best we can and making our lives good and providing for our families, there are often emotional blockages that prevent us from living the best life we can live. These blockages keep the path to the happiest version of ourselves closed off from our present selves, and they keep us away from doing what makes us the most content. The blockages in our lives can come in many forms, and they can affect every part of our lives. The fear of failure, fear of authority, the laziness we sometimes feel when we don't feel like we can keep going through our daily routine—all these things pile up on top of us and, if they aren't vented properly, they can pose a massive issue to our mental health and the way we live our lives. One of these blockages is usually some kind of anxiety. The crushing weight on our chest that makes it feel like we can't do anything that we'll never be good enough that we'll never be unique enough, and everything else we feel and think in the darkest part of our mind. The fear of inadequacy is disturbingly common in people who work busy lives, people who work with technology, or in-office jobs. Sometimes the rut we dig ourselves into compounds on us all at once, and we can't help but feel suffocated by our own choices and the circumstances we have put ourselves in. Anxiety is a beast, if only because it's so difficult to uproot from our lives, but when we can take hold of it and get a handle on it independently, we can shift our lives into a much healthier path—one which is calmer and more collected, not filled with the panic and anxiety that we might be used to.

One of the many issues that can arise from stress, anxiety, and depression is also one of the most common reasons that so many people tend to overthink—when we overthink, we spend all of our time thinking over the possible outcomes of an event and little time planning for those events. Because of this, we procrastinate, and we very rarely find the motivation to get out of our own heads and do the things we've been thinking about for days, maybe even weeks. One of the most significant issues with overthinking is that it feels as though we've done so much of the work anyway. When we spend so much of our time pouring over some of the possibilities of a decision we've already made, it can be daunting to think about acting on the decisions or the thoughts we have about them. In addition, we often psyche ourselves out of action when we overthink about the decision or our options going forward. When we dote on the choices we've made and the troubles we're probably going to have in the future because of those decisions, it can be challenging to get out of our own head and act on them. Though it's essential to think through our choices and weigh our options, there's usually a time where thinking about the decisions, things we could have done, and regrets we have about the decision, become effectively useless. At that point, we only become more stressed out the more than we think about the decision. When we feel so stressed out about our choices and our responsibilities that we stop acting on the pressure to complete tasks, we put them off to a nonexistent "better time". We imagine that, at a later point in time, we'll have calmed down and be much more able to take care of the problems we just can't seem to deal with right now. The reality is that this "better time" never really exists on its own. The best way to deal with procrastination is just by doing the thing that we're putting off. We often feel daunted by large tasks or things we have to do that feel too great, too large, too long, also essential for us to handle entirely on our own. This can make us feel isolated, alone, anxious, and depressed at the thought of failing with this project or chore we have to complete. Even if the thing we have to do or see or experience isn't particularly essential or stressful, poor time-management skills can also contribute to having a problem with chronic procrastination. Ultimately, it becomes more and more stressful and challenging to deal with issues, the longer we put them off. This becomes a cycle of stress where we put something off because we don't know how to function or deal with the stress of it, but the stress of the task ahead only grows faster and faster the more we put it off. Plus, the longer we put off a task, the more likely it is that more projects and chores will begin to pile up on top of the first task. We also put off these other tasks until we can finish the first one, and it becomes a giant list or a giant ball of things we need to do, things we beat ourselves up over not doing, but that we still don't do because we can't find the willpower just to do them and get them over with without thinking about it too much. Procrastination is a coping mechanism for some people who don't know how to deal with large amounts of stress or anxiety, but it's a coping mechanism that can destroy your way of life if you don't keep it under control or find ways to keep still completing essential tasks in your daily life.

There are many different ways that our habits of overthinking can manifest in our lives. There are also many different ways that these unhealthy habits can ruin us and break down our daily way of life. The critical thing to remember is that these negative feelings and habits are all temporary if we make the decision to put an end to them and get the help we may need if we want to be mentally stable and emotionally centered. When you feel overwhelmed by your negative emotions, it might be a good idea to take a step back from them and consider what changes you can try and make to your daily life to improve your overall experience.

CHAPTER 5:

Self-Chatter, Fears and Doubts

Where Self-Chatter Comes From

The result of psychotherapy can be assessed according to the degree of independence achieved by a person who has completed the relevant course. One of the most effective ways that people can help themselves is to encourage their own constructive changes through self-chatter that is, uttering specific phrases to themselves. Indeed, studies show that the nature of self-chatter becomes one of the most essential factors in case of problematic behavior, in particular, in the presence of social fears.

What is self-chatter?

Self-chatter is a series of phrases that we speak to ourselves. This is usually done very quickly, almost without stopping, especially when something takes our attention very much. This happens in several cases. 1) Before any action or event occurs. 2) During an activity or event. 3) After an activity or event. This internal dialogue expresses our perception of events, our pattern of behavior, judgments, habits, critical attitudes, desires, fears, and so on.

For example, someone comes to get a job. His self-chatter maybe this: "I would love to get this job, but no doubt there are more competent people than me. If I am asked questions that I cannot answer, everyone will understand that I am an idiot. I probably shouldn't have come to this interview. I do not have enough experience. I'm nervous, and everyone around is noticing. I stutter when I'm nervous and look ridiculous." This type of self-chatter only increases a person's social fears and reduces their capabilities.

How It Links to Self-Worth and Self-Esteem

Very often, self-chatter stops us or prevents us from doing something not so much our real inability, but rather (and more often) that we are not aware of our actual abilities and exaggerate our weaknesses. The study, which compared groups of people with high and low levels of social anxiety, revealed that people from a group with a high level of anxiety underestimate the positive results of their activities and overestimate the negative aspects. Their memory longer retains negative information, throwing out positive. In other words, it actually lowers our self-esteem and decreases our self-worth.

It seems rather apparent that the lack of self-esteem and social fears lead, among other things, to irrational expectations that manifest themselves in our self-chatter. Almost unconsciously, people with social anxiety tell themselves that in a given situation they will not know what to do, they will provoke a catastrophe, and others around them will turn away and so on.

How Understanding Our Fears Helps with Overthinking

Our own fears sometimes prevent us from defending our interests and fully communicating with others. And when we have no opportunity for self-assertion, we begin to feel incompetent and incapable. And the more we feel our incompetence, the more social anxiety increases, depriving us of the opportunity for self-assertion. Thus, a vicious circle arises. In this circle, there are three elements that are closely related. The first is social anxiety, the second is the lack of self-affirmation and communication, the third is a feeling of incompetence.

The objective reality is that we cannot both be alarmed and relaxed at the same time, but we can very easily learn how to deal with anxiety — learn how to relax. Numerous experimental studies show that relaxation can be useful for controlling stress and reducing vulnerability in stressful situations.

The ability to relax implies that we are able to recognize that we are tense. Therefore, it is essential to identify tangible voltage signals, to pay attention to what we feel. You can, for example, determine whether you are tense or relaxed at the moment. Are your hands tense? And the back? Do you have lower back pain? In the stomach? Does the headache? All this may be a sign that you are tense. Is your neck relaxed? And shoulders raised? Are the jaws clenched? If you are tense, you are overloading your body. Therefore, it is essential to pay attention to the stress that your body is experiencing and to relax as soon as you feel it.

The contrast of tension and relaxation will make you feel the difference between these two states. In addition, the tension of a particular muscle group helps you to be more attentive to what is happening in this part of your body in different situations.

How Doubting Yourself Affects Your Thoughts

Doubting yourself impacts many aspects of your life. Doubting produces irrational thoughts. Here are some examples of irrational thoughts:

"I would love to call Zhinnet, but if she doesn't call me herself, then she doesn't want to talk to me."

"I would like to have dinner at the restaurant with Paul, but if I myself offer it to him, he will think that I am imposing."

"If I tell the children that I want to be alone, they will think that I no longer love them."

We ourselves thus provoke the emergence of our anxiety when we say something like that, instead of thinking of how to resolve the situation. This leads to the fact that we strive to avoid situations that can cause social anxiety, and in fact only provoke an increase in our anxieties. Further, in these situations, we continue to see only the negative and do not notice the positive aspects. And besides, avoiding these situations, we are depriving ourselves of the opportunity to check how everything would be in reality. But perhaps we can reduce our worries by eliminating irrational and defeatist thoughts, replacing them with rational thoughts.

During an alarming situation, you can tell yourself the following phrases.

- I am calm, I continue to relax.
- If I overcome this situation step by step, I can handle it.
- I always think about what I can do and what positive events can happen.
- My tension can be my ally, because if I feel anxiety, then for me it serves as a signal that I must turn around to face the situation.
- I don't need to prove anything to anyone. If those around me accept, it is excellent, if not, then there is no need for the whole world to be my friends.
- I take a deep breath and relax. Everything is fine. I control the situation and myself.
- I am focused on the current situation. What can I do?
- It is possible that my fear increases, but it does not matter, I can relax and control its level.

- I perfectly capture what is happening around me. During this time, I do not think about my anxieties.

When an alarming situation is completed, the following phrases will allow you to maintain a sense of self-confidence and a feeling of success.

- I achieved success.
- It was better than I could have imagined.
- If I can control my thoughts, then I can manage my fear.
- I am pleased with my own progress. I will tell this to my best friend.

You can choose from these phrases those that you find most useful, or find others.

Ways to Stop Doubting Yourself

We will build a hierarchy of our fears, defining those social situations that cause us to doubt ourselves, then those that cause average anxiety, then those that cause extreme anxiety. Here is an example of a hierarchy built on observing your fears.

1. I walk down the street and greet the neighbor.

2. I walk down the street; the postman caught up with me and greeted me.

3. I walk down the street, and a group of five people greets me.

4. I am waiting for the bus, and people are looking at me at the bus stop.

BOB LIPTON & LISA MACALLEN PHD

5. I am going to buy a liter of milk at the grocery store. At the exit, I pass by a group of people who are looking at me.

As you can see in these examples of hierarchies, the first scenes cause a little alarm, the last scenes cause severe anxiety, and the middle scenes cause a middle alarm. After these explanations and these examples, you can probably build your own hierarchy of fears.

Exercise

Make a list. On it, there are twelve positions for describing social situations that cause you concern. Describe each scene, giving all the details about the people who took part in it, about the place, about the relationship, about the behavior of people and so on. Fixing the details will help you find the least exciting scenes by changing these details (for example, speaking to the public from one hundred and fifty spectators, fifty spectators, twenty spectators, ten spectators, and so on).

Under number one, describe the social situation that is causing you some slight anxiety, and at number twelve - describe the social condition that causes an extreme concern. Then find the situations between these two extremes and arrange them in order of increasing anxiety from lesser to higher. Your description of these scenes should be specific enough so that you can easily imagine them. In addition, the degree of anxiety should gradually increase by a small amount from one scene to another.

Now that you have built your own hierarchy of fears, assess your level of anxiety in each of these situations on a scale from zero to one hundred, where zero means no anxiety, and one is the point of maximum anxiety or even panic. Put your score from zero to one hundred next to each of the scene descriptions. It is essential that you build your hierarchy so that the difference in estimates of neighboring

39 | P a g .

scenes does not exceed ten to fifteen points, in other words, there should not be too much difference in the estimates of one after other scenes.

The practice of visualization: first, you need to try this practice yourself. Imagine or remember a specific situation. This allows you better to visualize each of the scenes in your hierarchy.

Stay as comfortable as possible, for example, lying or sitting in a comfortable chair. Then close your eyes and imagine pleasant scenes for you. For example, an evening on the river bank, a village or a ski resort ... To your personal taste. Imagine this scene clearly, with all the essential details. Try not to be distracted from this scene. Present it as if you are present in it, rather than looking at it from the side. You are a member of this scene. You see objects, people, you hear sounds, you touch things, people, and you experience emotions as if you were there.

To help yourself more accurately, imagine your presence in that situation, ask yourself the questions: "In the place where I am, what do I see and what do I hear? Where are the other people? What emotions do they express, how tall are they, what are their voices? What am I thinking about? What do I say to others? I want to eat or drink? What does my body feel?"

Imagine this scene for about two minutes. Then relax. Forget this situation, focus only on relaxation. Then again, remember this scene for another two minutes. Relax again.

If you have difficulties with the presentation of this situation, you can start by performing the following exercise. Look at some object or person. Then close your eyes and imagine this object or this person.

CHAPTER 6:

Where Does Overthinking Come from and Why Does it Happen?

Where Does Overthinking Come from?

Wh\hat comes into your mind when you hear of over thinking? Do you visualize a physical clutter that you know of? Overthinking simply means mental overload, mental stress or mental fatigue. This is anything that gives you anxiety, depression, frustration, sense of overwhelm, and anger. This comes in the form of:

- Regrets for past failures and regret for not doing some things that you should have done
- Too many bills to pay and increasing debts as well as unfinished projects
- Worries and insecurities
- Inner critic
- Feeling bad for failing to achieve something

These thoughts hinder us from focusing and working to improve ourselves. They divert our thoughts to the past instead of focusing on now and tomorrow. Overthinking occupies our mental space, messes with our minds, eliminates our mental clarity and it is bad for our mental health.

How Can Over Thinking Lead to Unrealistic Scenarios?

Due to Someone's Behavior or a Comment Made in The Past

We should take responsibility for our wrongdoings and learn some lessons from it. Never allow yourself to be a prisoner of guilt and shame in the past because it will cause you to have resentment self-hate, and even kill your self-esteem. The best way to get rid of guilt and shame is to acknowledge your mistake, forgive yourself and move on. This will empower you, motivate you to become a better person, make you value yourself. You should never repeat the same mistake.

A person's mind usually picks up on negative experiences from the past because the experiences went contrary to the person's expectations. However, if things went according to plan, then the thoughts become happy memories.

Due to Something You Don't Understand

Overthinking about things you don't understand without actually doing them is a waste of time, primarily if fear and worry motivate the person.

How do you perceive yourself? Do you frequently have negative self-talk dominating your mind because of something you don't understand? Negative self-talk will limit our mental growth and lower our self-confidence. Remember your brain will believe what you tell it. If you continuously tell yourself that you cannot do it, your mind will act according to that belief.

You need to learn to refuse negative self-talk and replace it with positive talk. If the inner critic is telling you that you cannot do it then do it and you will silence that inner critic that is hindering your progress in life.

Due to Something You don't know How to Address

When we encounter challenges in our daily activities, our brains naturally go to a state of worry. Although it is a natural reaction, we can always control it because it will not solve any of our problems. Instead, worrying will worsen the situation. Worrying will take away your peace of mind and it will stress you. Worrying is a waste of energy.

The best thing you can do is to stop worrying. Find something to do that will divert your thoughts to something better like going for a walk, dancing, cooking or anything that interests you. You can also write down those things that are robbing you of your peace of mind and write how you are going to solve them.

Due to Something You are Confused About

What if' situations are useful when a person is confused about different outcomes of certain risk factors.

Confusion is an enemy of progress! You should not allow fear to hinder you from taking chances and chasing after your dreams and enjoying life. Do you dream of owning a business but you are afraid that it might not take off if you start? Start it anyway and silence the fear that you have.

Overthinking About the Opinion of Others

Gee whiz! "I wish I worked hard in school my life could be better!" Such remarks are common when having a conversation with friends or family members. We all have those things we wish we had done or not done in our lives! Sometimes our minds can focus on those things but we should not allow it. Focusing your minds on regrets will rob you of your happiness and cause you mental fatigue and stress. You cannot change the past so put your energy into creating a better vision for your life.

There is no way you can be happy with being so affected to the opinion of others. It will bring you feelings of anger, sadness, discontent and it will be hard for you to have positive feelings like being happy, confident or proud. The overthinking will spike your stress hormones giving you dull feelings every day.

When your mind is full of clutter, you will not be able to receive new ideas because there is not any room left for them. Your life will only be revolving around the clutter in your mind that are usually worries from past events and uncertainty of the future. Whining about your past situations will derail you from achieving a better tomorrow. So let go of your past and have a clear plan of how you can make your aspirations and goals in life.

The Difference between Objective Statements and Opinions

An objective is a goal, but to be objective means to be impartial. When it is objective to you, you don't have any personal opinions about it. When someone tells us something that somehow hurt our feelings, we should learn to evaluate the situation. Was it a mere opinion or an objective statement? This is then the time for us to understand that these statements should be taken positively to make us a better version of ourselves.

How Too Much Information Can Overcharge Your Brain

Too much information promotes stress and anxiety that will suck your energy making you feel lazy, unproductive, and useless. It will distract your focus because so many things are fighting for your attention and this can affect your productivity. Having an endless "to-do" list can be hard to handle and it can make you feel like you are losing your mind.

This feeling of never completing projects will ground your mind and it will create negative self-talk that can hinder your progress.

When your mind is full, you may find that you do not remember where you put specific files then you spend so much time looking for those work files. These can delay your work, you may fail to meet deadlines, and this may make you feel like giving up.

Overthinking will prevent you from processing relevant information. It can also lead to temporary memory loss. Overthinking will take away your focus leaving you confused with endless "to-do" tasks. Such overwhelming feelings will render you helpless and you may find that even doing a small task is difficult. It can also affect your parenting styles negatively because you will project your anger and frustration on the children and that is not good for their mental growth.

Symptoms or Typical Behaviors of An Over thinker

You are Always Stressed

When you have an endless list of unfinished projects, unpaid bills, and debts, it can lead to stress. Mental clutter will stress the brain and it will release a stress hormone cortisol. This can lead to some undesirable health conditions like chronic stress, high blood pressure, slow digestion, poor sleeping habits, and depression that can cause mental illness.

Stress will exhaust your mental energy leaving you feeling tired and overwhelmed. It will also make you lose focus and concentration on important things and it promotes negative self-talk.

You have unhealthy eating habits

Mental clutter can make you lose appetite or crave for more unhealthy food because of the rise of stress levels. Research has shown that people with mental clutter eat twice as many cookies, sweets, and snacks than those people who do not suffer from mental clutter. That means when you have a mental clutter you will not prioritize a healthy diet but you will crave junk food, which is unhealthy and it can make you fat.

You don't have peace of mind

Your mind can never relax if you are suffering from mental clutter. It will always be wandering! This will leave you with stress, frustration, discontent, and these feelings can be overwhelming to your mind. Find something that can help you decongest your mind and relax. You can listen to soothing music, meditate or take a walk in the park, anything that will relieve your mental clutter.

You always procrastinate

Since mental clutter will drain your energy, you will end up postponing some tasks because of mental fatigue and stress. The best way to stop procrastination is by clearing your mind of unnecessary thoughts so that it can focus on doing important things that can make you a better person.

You can't manage money effectively

Mental clutter can cause you to have surprise bills because you may have forgotten to pay them. The clutter in your mind may make you forget to pay bills on time and this can cause you to pay some penalty fee. It can also cause you to have bad credits. You may also find yourself buying stuff that you already have but you cannot remember. Mental clutter can also make you forget to keep count of how much money you use per week or month and this will make you a poor financial manager.

You seem not to get promoted no matter how hard you try

When you lose focus and concentration in your work, you become less productive and this is not healthy for your career. Most managers demand performance in the workplace and you cannot keep up with that if you have mental clutter. If you want to be successful in your career, you need to clear your mind and focus on doing your best in everything you do.

Self-Evaluation for an Over thinker

If you question if overthinking is an issue for yourself, answer the questions below to evaluate yourself.

- Were you conscious at a particular given point in time about what you think?
- Would you ask yourself sometimes why do you have these ideas?
- Do you sometimes search for the greater understanding of your thinking or their deep significance?
- Have you ever reflected about what you thought once you're feeling frustrated?
- Would you have a deep desire to learn or understand the complexities of your imagination?
- Would you think it is critical that you must have absolute control over the situation?
- Have you had a weak resistance to intrusive, spontaneous thoughts?
- Do you still find yourself struggling to manage your thoughts?

Now, evaluate yourself. You may have a potential to overthink if you replied yes to several of these questions.

CHAPTER 7:

Overthinking Your Relationship

Acknowledge Who You Are and Why You Want a Relationship

We should grab the chance to develop tremendously emotionally and personally with your mate or potential partner. It is only through this partnership that you are able to understand to become more empathetic and present.

You will be in a position to know how you would like your connection to develop in the future. Remember there will always be no perfect relationship. There are still some defects in your mate. Never adequately fulfill all the standards you have in your imagination.

Instead of turning to someone else to improve relationships, the great place to begin is inside yourself. Even though your close relatives, colleagues, and business contacts have to develop their interpersonal skills, by making improvements within you, you will go a bit of a way in minimizing tension in your existence. People cannot influence anything either — you only have the ability to monitor whether you communicate with people next to you and whether you respond to them.

Paradoxically, our interactions with love try to regard us with the hardest problems of our lives, likely to cause the most "anxious thoughts" and discomfort. Exercising your love life awareness gives you a technique for enhancing your romantic bond while raising tension and anxiety in your daily existence.

If you can override your spouse's emotional responses, you become better focused, relaxed and able to solve conflicts in a caring way. That strength itself will help you survive moments and perhaps even months of psychological and emotional depression which is depleting your personal neediness.

Deciding not to go on the deck is the start of a mindful partnership which helps to restore bonding instead of conflict and disunity.

Overthinking Perfectionism

There is no such thing as perfect. The person you imagine your partner to be, is not the same person in the real life. We all have an ideal type of person in mind. It may be someone caring, loving, and a not jealous kind of person. Bear in mind that you should always be open to new possibilities. We should learn how to lower our expectation for us not to be disappointed in the long run.

Comparison creates far too many painful thoughts that now it ruins more than just your sense of security — it harms your partnerships. The further you dwell on whether you conform, chronic stress you think in yourself and the other individual. Selfishness, resentment, humiliation, remorse, humiliation, self-loathing, disappointment, and frustration are not attributes that strengthen a bond or makes you desirable to anyone else.

Such impulses can escalate very quickly, trying to make us feel terrible towards ourselves whereas perceiving others as the source of our sadness. Through weighing ourselves against someone else's successes, properties or attributes, we laid the foundation for the breakdown of possibly satisfying relationships.

It takes mental energy to disconnect from contrast and the feelings that follow it. Yet shifting your responses to others who have "more" would give you freedom to pursue your own course and be the right person to be.

Have Realistic Expectations

How could partnerships add much more to our satisfaction, yet still be an immense cause of psychological stress? The trick is not to just have relationships — it has common goals with each other. Both partnerships warrant effort and collaboration. We each have our own shortcomings which we seek to strengthen daily. Either you're with a long-term partner, colleague, friend or relative or maybe even a work companion, a long-lasting relationship should contain:

- Making relationships a priority
- Opening up social interaction
- A sustainable agreement to clashes
- Confidence and cooperation
- Mutual common values
- Any degree of mental and/or physical affection
- Sympathy and reconciliation
- Direct contact (for intimate intercourse)

Engagement is a decision to be developed daily. For personal health and contentment, it is essential to build, sustain and cultivate positive relationships.

It's hard to afford attention to things, when our heads are loaded of far too many emotions. That when somebody talks, our brain is much more concentrated on the meticulousness of our situations, our problems, or what we'd like to share next.

Understanding Yourself and Your Thoughts

Conscientiousness is also the first step towards improvement. For particular for your romantic relationship, we suggest paying careful attention to the words during a conversation. Establish a barrier from your words and thoughts and understand the impact your actions have on one of your life's biggest people.

You should first be mindful with your thoughts for you to understand yourself better. You will then realize why and how you acted those ways in your relationship. For example, if you laugh a lot in your relationship, this means that your thoughts and your mind is also releasing positive thoughts.

Fight the urge to respond easily to statements or acts of others. Pause a second to select your terms deliberately. Converse in caring, compassionate, and polite terms and seek to use a calm, non - aggressive tone, mainly if the other individual is upset or irritated.

When you talk more attentively, everyone around you also will react courteously. You are motivating yourself to retain self-control and personal fulfillment, even though they don't.

You also strengthen the quality of the relationship, but also enhance the consistency of your internal self through all the process of conscious expression.

No level of reflection, quibbling, and fixating will affect who you really are, how much you have achieved, and whatever you actually own. The individual you are for is now everything that you have, just for a bit.

Take a step on it, instead of restraining that person. Recognize that, and admit that right here you are perfectly okay. It's freeing and inspiring only to embrace this feeling of revolutionary self-acceptance.

How an Over thinker Can Apply Unfair Expectations

How much do you find yourself annoyed, upset or even angry with your friends and family?

The response to this question is essential since difficulties with relationships have become a contributing source of suffering which partners feel in life.

As an over thinker, you sometimes feed too much negative thoughts in your mind. Without you knowing it, you are already expecting too much in someone. It may be because, inside our minds, we recreate awkward experiences and obsess over such a minor transgression over hours. And we're separated from our family and friends, just to feel anxious, alienated and unappreciated.

People construct distorted cognitive impressions about specific people, attaching behavior and feelings to them which might or might not be valid but that nevertheless feel insulting and intimidating.

Whereas the significant people may be the cause of mental discomfort, our personal relations are one of the essential aspects of life that contribute to long-term fulfillment.

What does a Healthy Relationship Look Like?

A healthy relationship requires a lot of hard work. Unless there is an ongoing issue or injure to both you and this other person, speak up to fix the conflict. Instead of simmering over the past issue, initiate communication with the other person to talk through all of it, even though you believe that you have been correct. It's indeed impossible to obtain out to those who have harmed you, but the inconvenience of doing something like this is much less than the delayed agony of festering over painful feelings.

Some of the reconciliation may include expressing your emotions and frustration, responding to the viewpoint of the other person, seeking or saying sorry and considering the current relationship future. Remove the bind of the past experience from inside through thinking freely about all this.

People will never confess to the individual from the history but give forgiveness nevertheless. People may not have to accept them personally, but pardon them within your own soul and spirit. Trying to cling to the frustration and misery just lengthens the emotional anguish and suffering. People absolve to release oneself from that kind of pain, so that you might carry on with a positive mindset to deal with reality.

The Importance of Communication in a Relationship

The desire to become more attentive towards your mate is not based on the mutual interest of your relationship-but it helps enormously.

Take a seat and then let your partner know regarding your new strategy, if you can speak without disruption. You could suggest anything like that, "I realized I needed to become more caring and far more involved in my partnership towards you. This will bring us together and allow us to overcome our conflicts despite having too much frustration or damage. I made a vow to all this, and if you'd agree to it too, I would also like to."

Once you have a disagreement or highly emotional argument with your partner, participation includes listening before planning your reply or defense.

Being mindful of your inner responsive feelings, label those and accept why they were activated, and don't behave upon them. Seek to bring the focus back to the language of your spouse, then understand that the feelings of your spouse are just as relevant with your own.

Change course to the process of healing once you have a problem with your partner, instead of just taking a dig at them and then creating a derogatory statement. Look out for your thoughts and feelings and sit tight till you're relaxed and far less protective before you initiate a discussion.

Address the matter beyond reproach or critique. Comment your understanding of the problem, how everything makes you feel a bit and also what your relationship wants to re-establish your bond. Respond to the answer and viewpoint from your spouse without being hostile.

Techniques for a Healthy Relationship

There are countless ways to know if you want a healthy relationship. These four techniques will guide you build a healthy one.

1. Convey consistent appreciation.

Comparisons make us indifferent to everything we have. We get so concentrated to the other person and how we wouldn't match up that we all don't notice all the benefits within us.

It's about having the bottle half full instead of quarter unused — and recognizing your appreciation for the liquid in the bottle.

2. Create the promise.

With the knowledge that awareness will boost the value of your current relationship, dedicate yourself every day to practice this behavior.

Whether you have spent so many years in an implicit partnership that is responsive to both you and your spouse, it will take a bit of time to reskill yourself to communicate differently. Yet if you've been inspired to develop and overcome stress in your future, you can adapt.

3. Stay mentally engaged.

To be emotionally stable requires being entirely committed for interaction with your spouse. When your spouse is in distress it requires openness to the discomfort mentally and having empathy.

4. Despite disruption, enjoy spending around him/her.

Every time also engaged partners need to plan since situations are exhausting and stressful. If that is indeed the situation for you, point out the irony of scheduling a casual outing with your partner, or just 20 minutes of occasional relaxation place, in which you can chat and reconcile.

CHAPTER 8:

Thinking Your Life Purpose or Career

How do you maintain your organizational skills and evolve into the future? What are your long-term goals and dreams? Do you want to be healthier? Do you want to advance in your career? Have more robust relationships with your spouse or family? You might wish to acquire new skills. Whatever it is that you see yourself moving towards, we will help you set and keep those goals

How to Break Down Your Interests and Passion

What are your core interests and passion? Have you ever taken the time to write them down and examine them? If you have done so in the past, are you still that person, or have your life changed? To turn it around a bit, is it the things you value that have changed? When you have a solid concept of your interests and passion, you'll be able to march into the future with a clear mind and new confidence.

Some of us are born talented, while some develop their skills through time. Even there have been cases when you recognize your own desire, but sadly, the circumstances prohibit that you develop those talents and passion. Some are lucky to be able to pursue their deepest dreams. However, other people have no choice but strive hard and do what is available for them to do because of life's obstacles. In this life, we have a freedom to choose what path we will going to take. We should make sure we make the most of it.

Acknowledging Your Skills and What You Need to Work On

Acknowledging your skills means being able to know what are your best interests and at the same time evaluating the skills that you lack knowledge on. If you asked your friends or coworkers to describe you, what would their answers be? Would they be the same as yours or very different?

Being able to identify these skills can guide you into your future, because you can use them when you are making decisions. Your values will play into what type of career you choose and who you look to when making friends or seeking romantic partners. You'll want to associate yourself with others who have similar values and skills to avoid unnecessary conflict. It's only when you have defined a well-rounded set of values and skills for yourself that you can begin to craft your future.

Realizing False Beliefs about What You Can Achieve

When you've discovered your skills and defined your values, and found a hobby you are passionate about, what's to say that you cannot combine all aspects of your life and turn your avocation into a vocation? Several people have come across means of transforming interests into business ventures, and side businesses into their primary income. There's just no ceiling to what you can do!!

Maybe you've done some work for a charity organization and realized there is a greater need for services in your immediate area. You could start your own foundation with the purpose of filling that need. The point is, where you are now doesn't define where you will end up, and if you want things to change, you need to make that change for yourself, your family, and your community. If you really are able to attain them, there are resources everywhere around us.

Perhaps you are already working in your dream job, but you want more- a promotion, to further your company's message, to find a way to give back. Use your platform to raise your voice. Professional athletes and other celebrities do it all the time. It's all about creating your personal brand and using it to make life better for yourself and others. Decide who you want to be and present yourself as such at all times. Find a signature piece of clothing or jewelry, or a catchphrase or motto. These things will help you become recognizable in your community and beyond.

While it's essential to find a job or career path that fits in well with your values and the person you are and want to be, it's also really crucial to have a passion or hobby outside of your work. Do you have a charitable cause that you believe in? You can find ways to get involved in your community to support that cause. You can find service organizations in every corner of the world that give back to others and promote social equality.

Perhaps you are really good with your hands, and you'd like to take up woodworking or other craftsmanship. Do it! You could still find some people of same opinion across the web and in your community, who share that passion. You'll find advice, be able to purchase inexpensive secondhand tools to get started, and you'll make new friends. Life is hectic, and making time for hobbies is critical for good mental health and overall wellbeing.

You could find hobbies that you can take up with your children to spend more quality time together. People of all ages can enjoy hiking and camping, and fresh air never hurt anyone. Find a 'mommy and me' dance or music class or an open volleyball league that you can play in with older children. What counts most at the end of each day is that you make time for things you love with the people that you love.

Places to Look to Build Skills and Improve Career Paths

If you are searching to   have effective leadership or developing oneself, here are a   few   fantastic opportunities to learn the vital skills that will make your life easier.

1. Life hacker

Life hacker is the tool to practice how to do something easier, quicker and more intelligently.

2. Library of Congress

Most of the text from our central archives is accessible online now. Whichever expertise you wish to know, there you can give it a read

3. Boundless

Recall taking on a new part-time job only to provide for those textbooks in college? Boundless is completely changing the instructional industry by implementing digital textbooks, free of charge.

4. TED Talks

TED would be another right place to enjoy realistic recommendations and opportunities for learning that actual, professional people make.

5. YouTube

YouTube contains billions of videos that will help you in everything you want to do in life. This social media platform is a perfect tool for learning online tutorials about the different courses and skills that will help you improve your talents.

Make the most of social networks; this can be a powerful platform when used correctly. You can build a following for your business or charity, spread the word about events and occasions, and make new connections. Use your goal-setting skills to define milestones you'd like to hit in your personal and professional life. When you have a strongly defined purpose, you'll be better able to withstand setbacks, battle mental clutter, and reach your goals on time.

Mind Mapping

When you set goals, it's essential to understand the short-term and long-term needs for everything you want to accomplish. You can lay them out on paper to create a visual representation of your full timeline and the steps necessary to achieve your goals. To get you started, use the sheet below as a template.

Goal: _____

Target date: _____

Step One: _____

Target date: _____

Tasks: _____

_____

_____

Step Two: _____

Target date: _____

Tasks: _____

_____

_____

Step Three: _____

Target date: _____

Tasks: _____

_____

_____

Misc. Considerations: _____

Then, you can list all of your potential talents and skills in a table form like this one below:

Talent/Skill to be Developed	Long Term/ Short Term Goal	Target Date to Master the Skill
Design Thinking	Long Term	May 2021

Communication Skills	Long Term	Feb 2021
Attention to Detail	Short Term	October 2020

Example of a Skills Mind Map

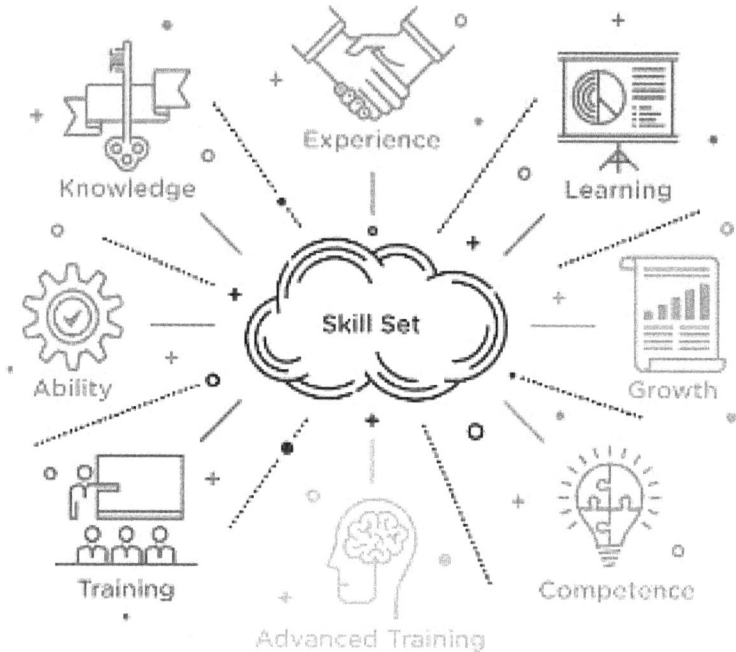

My Passion and My Future Goals: What I Value

Your values are the principles that you live your life by and by which you base your decisions. Think about the things that are important to you, especially the things you are not willing to compromise. These are things like loyalty, honesty, strong work ethic, and/or integrity in business and in love. You want to think about how you present yourself to the world and how you make choices around those values.

Values can also be a set of personal beliefs, like faith in your religion or your politics. Your values can also encompass the material items you find necessary to live your life in the fashion you desire. This could be your sense of fashion, how you choose to decorate your living space, or what type of car you prefer to drive. All these things make up the core of who you are. Make a list of your values and evaluate whether you're currently living your life up to your own standards. If you're not, how can you attain those values or get back to them if you've drifted away?

Having a robust set of values can guide you into your future, because you can use them when you are making decisions. Your values will play into what type of career you choose and who you look to when making friends or seeking romantic partners. You'll want to associate yourself with others who have similar values to avoid unnecessary conflict. It's only when you have defined a well-rounded set of values for yourself that you can begin to craft your future.

Keeping a journal is one way to maintain your values. How, you might ask? People are never more true or honest than when they are talking to themselves. A journal is a regular record of your thoughts and feelings, hopes, and dreams. When you scribble or doodle in a journal, you are expressing how you feel in the exact same moment that your pen hit the paper. If that's not a reflection of your inner self and true values, there are not too many other things that could come closer.

CHAPTER 9:

Rebalance Yourself

What Creates Imbalance

The ghost of the past is tough to go. This is one of the most significant causes of imbalance in our lives. The harder we try to push it, the more resounding it gets. It comes to haunt at the most inconvenient times. It should come as no surprise that you always remember everything bad that has happened in your life. Your mind is a terrific storage device. It has unlimited storage ability. Scientists believe that you can record more than 2.5 petabytes of data in your brain and still have space left for more. It actually translates to 300 million hours of video recording space. This is huge.

It means that all the things that have happened in your life, positive or negative, are recorded in your mind. However, your mind also has a strong response to negative things as it feels the need to keep playing them, again and again, to keep you safe from falling into the same kind of situation. It is a survival mechanism designed for good.

The problem begins when your mind starts playing the negative things obsessively and makes it impossible for you to start fresh. It makes wiping the slate clean tough. Your mind clutter has a vital role to play in this. You let your past remain heavy on you. The solace of victimhood, the desperation to stay safe and vulnerability are some of the strong reasons. These feelings encroach your productive space. They leave no room for positive thinking.

This all happens because you are not being mindful. You have allowed your mind to remain cluttered by negative experiences and want to be in a safe sanctuary.

If you let your mind and thoughts rule your world then you will rot in a corner without ever seeing the light of the day. It will keep telling you that the world is full of dangers and risks.

Too Much Thinking Paralyses Us

If you have failed at something, your mind will trigger nervousness whenever you get in a similar situation. Suppose you failed at one job interview. Your mind will make you nervous whenever you go for the next interview. It will keep telling that you'll fail as you had failed the last time. Your mind is not thinking clearly. It is full of the past baggage of failure. You will have to clear your mind of such thoughts and remind yourself of your merits for the position.

Remind yourself that you came for the interview as you thought yourself capable for the job. You have the abilities and therefore, there is no reason to be so sure of failure even this time. Your failure in the past interview can have several causes. Also if it was your inability to answer some questions, the required thing to do is to work on that part and not to worry about the results. You must make your mind understand that only action is in your hand. The consequences of the actions are beyond your control and therefore they are none of your business.

An overthinking mind will keep invoking these fears. It will keep your judgment shrouded. It will never let you see clearly. Its instincts are to keep you safe. It builds a safe sanctuary for you. However, it will take you nowhere. You will have to begin reasoning. Rational thinking doesn't mean you need to take unnecessary risks but it means taking calculated risks. When you take calculated risks, you know the amount of fall you can take and you are already prepared for that. You are ready for it.

The Role of Your Relationship with Others in Maintaining the Balance

Live in the moment. Your friends, family, relationship and career are also essential factors in maintaining balance in your life.

These relationships are essential in our lives. They give meaning to our existence. However, all relationships are not meant to last forever. For one reason or another people grow apart. Relationships do not remain cordial but your desires to be in them always remain the same. This desire is the cause of most of the troubles. A relationship which hasn't worked is not going to give you anything. If you harbor the desire to be in it, you'll be causing more pain and sorrow for yourself and the other person. Your mind would always remain occupied with planning to make things work.

We all need healthy relationships. Healthy relationships fill the void in our lives. They make us feel content. However, if we keep looking for relationships to make us happy, we'll keep feeling miserable. In that case, we become dependent on them. We give the charge of our happiness to the relationships. This is the beginning of the problems in the first place. Any relationship will only be fulfilling if you are there to contribute. The day you enter into a link to receive, you'll make it toxic. The joy and satisfaction of giving make the relationship happy.

We are emotional beings and therefore, we can easily get influenced by the outside world. However, overdependence on the outside world can take away all the happiness from our lives. The world is full of negativity and if you go looking for it, you'll strike gold.

What does a Well-Balanced Life Look Like?

We keep sulking about things. There is an endless pursuit of happiness and we continuously try to find it in one thing or the other. Think of all the moments of pure happiness and joy that you experienced in the last 24 hours. Ideally, your counting wouldn't go more than half a dozen if you are very positive. Some people might not be able to recall even one incident of happiness in the past 24 hours. Now, think of your childhood. It was a time when you had to be made unhappy forcefully. Unhappiness required an outward force. Joy and happiness came naturally to you. You never needed outside stimuli to be happy. You are still the same person. The only thing that has changed is your perception. Now, you have more in your plate than you can chew. You've got far too much on your head that you are never able to rejoice the moments of happiness or experience real joy.

We have become so preoccupied with ourselves that we have started taking this precious life for granted. We ignore all the precious blessings and keep searching for happiness outside. If happiness has to come, then it can only come from inside. You can only enjoy the tastiest food in the world in a real sense, only if you are happy. If you are happy, then even simple food will taste great. The same goes for everything else.

Real joy only comes when you find something that makes you happy. Find your calling in things like traveling, creative pursuits, and hobbies that make you happy. Only the inner joy of accomplishing something can make you truly happy.

Tips on How to Maintain Balance

Can't Undo Spilled Milk; Make Cheese Out of It

You can't remove negativity by negativity. If there is a problem, then brooding over it will not help. Think of the ways to overcome it.

On day to day basis, we come across several situations which have gone beyond our control. Crying over them will not help our cause. The only way to deal with such cases is to devise ways to nullify their effect. If you are late to work, then either choosing a fast transport could help or think of a better excuse. Brooding over getting late is not going to be of any help.

Stop Punishing Yourself

Negative thoughts are a torment. They lead to stress and anxiety. It is well known that stress and anxiety have a detrimental impact on your physiological as well as psychological health. They act as triggers that begin several negative processes. Your body starts releasing stress hormones that lead to fat accumulation, lethargy, and heartburn, stiffness in muscles and the works. Your body reacts poorly to these triggers.

Consciously Embrace Positivity

The negative thought process is very imposing. It has a powerful impact on your psyche. Merely trying to dodge this state will not help you. You'll need to make attempts to ensure the events will be lighter consciously. Positive things around you are beneficial in the process. Remove clutter around you. Organize your surroundings, as it also leads to negativity. Cherish your small accomplishments. These tiny steps to embrace positivity will help you in overcoming negative thought patterns.

Learn New Things

Learning is a very positive process. It fills your mind with positivity and new energy. When you are learning new things, your mind is focused on possibilities rather than limitations. It provides a great stimulus to the brain. If negative thought patterns keep troubling you, then learning new things can give you great relief. They are proving to be a big distraction from anxiety and stress. You get to use a more significant part of your mind and it stops thinking about negative things.

Engage Yourself in Physical Activity

The extent of physical activities carried out by us has gone down considerably. We mostly live a sedentary lifestyle tied down to chairs or our couches. There is a lot of mental activity and stress but we don't get enough physical activity. This imbalance also creates a lot of negativity. Indulge yourself in physical activities. Gardening, exercise, repair or things, or building something new are some of the activities that will challenge your body.

Creative Works

Creative pursuits like painting, drawing, playing some musical instruments are some of the activities that can help in distracting you from negative thoughts. They require you to exercise undivided attention. Your mind automatically drifts away from negative thoughts.

Deep Breathing Exercises

Breathing is a fundamental function. We breathe every moment. Yet we rarely consider the significance of this critical operation. Missing our breath for a couple of minutes can mean the end of all. Yet, this crucial process never gets our attention. If negative thoughts are not leaving your trail then deep breathing exercises can help you.

Long-term Effects of a Balanced Lifestyle

A balanced healthy lifestyle can carry benefits — either in the long and short term. Not only does the body look and feel healthier, but you'll have an increased standard of health, get less chance of sickness and therefore can continue to retire further than individual peers who don't follow a healthy lifestyle.

People have a lowered heart attack risk, internal bleeding, collapses and lacerations, diabetes, as well as hormonal imbalances which otherwise are becoming more harder to cure as people gets older. They are more expected to live healthier, and be satisfied and much more engaged than people who consume fewer nutritious diets.

CHAPTER 10:

How to Break the Habit of Overthinking

Replacing the Thought is The Key

There are different ways to break the habit of overthinking. One great solution is by replacing your negative thoughts with positive ones. Suppressing your thoughts and emotions will not be a good help. It will only worsen your situation. By suppressing it, you are feeding the negative emotions in your mind which will then trigger everything.

When it comes to your emotions, you need to ensure that you deal with them the right way without affecting the people around you. For you to deal with your feelings healthily, you need to understand that emotions are natural. That means expressing them is healthy, but you need a way of showing them the right direction. Adjusting your expectations is another way of dealing with your emotions healthily. You might feel frustrated or disappointed because you expect too much from others or yourself. For example, if you are a mother, you should not follow what others tell you to be a perfect mum, but you should be realistic.

Don't try to be perfect, but be a good mother as you can. Learning how to accept how things or people are a healthy way of dealing with your emotions. For example, if you don't like how your kid behaves, you need to accept that way. Instead of shouting at him, you can find the right way of communicating with him.

However, if it is hard for you to deal with your emotions by yourself, you can seek help from psychologists. They will help you to understand your feelings quickly and how to deal with them healthily.

How to Redirect Your Thinking through Self-Introspection

Having a negative emotion has many effects, especially on your health and people that surround you. Having a negative emotion can lead to health problems such as chronic stress. It can lead to a more serious health problem that shortens your life spun. Having a negative emotion can make you aggressive, and it will be hard for you to live with other people in peace. You will find that you are always angry and rude because you have a negative emotion. It will be impossible for you to be happy when you have a negative feeling, and most of the time, you will be sad.

A key to overcome these negative emotions is through self-introspection.

Redirecting your thoughts can be done through self-introspection. In this technique, you have to practice self-awareness and self-regulation.

Emotions are feelings composed in your thoughts, and they can be as a result of the situation that you are in or the people around you. It is possible to control your emotions by dealing with them intelligently and staying positive. Some of the emotions include happiness, anger, hatred, love, and fear.

Some of the situations that can arouse emotions include when you are in a sad or happy situation or when you are scared. The things that surround you or the ones you are thinking about can also arouse emotions. Being in a place where you are treated unfairly or fairly can arouse emotions or being in an uncomfortable situation.

Benefits of Letting Go

You get away from negative thoughts

You need to ensure that you get away from conditions that cause unwanted feelings. If you know that there is something that makes you angry or being in a particular situation, you should avoid them. For example, if you get mad when you are late to work, you can always make sure that you wake up early to avoid being late. If being around a particular person makes you frustrated or angry, it is better to avoid that person as much as possible.

You can modify the situation you are in

You might be feeling disappointed because you cannot do something in the right direction or as you aimed. You can reduce disappointment by finding a good way that you will do that thing the right way or as you expected. For example, you may be willing to prepare a nice meal for your family, but in the end, the feed does not please them. You can avoid the situation by finding a simple recipe on how to prepare that meal and be sure to make a meal that your family will love. In that way, you have modified the situation, and you will not be disappointed.

You can shift your emotions to the positive side

You might be in a situation where you feel inferior because of the people that are surrounding you because they are higher than you. For example, you can be a class group where you are the only one who is less intelligent. They know almost everything, and you keep admiring them and feeling sorry for you.

You can become socially intelligent

In that way, you will start feeling superior and feel confident about your intelligence. If possible, you can shift from that group and join another one where you will be able to focus on yourself. Through that process, you will start desiring your intelligence, and you won't feel inferior anymore.

You can easily change your thoughts

Everyone has beliefs that drive their emotions. One feels sad when something did not work as expected or when they lose a friend. You will also feel happy when something happens as you expected or when you are expecting something good in your life. When you change your thought, you will change how you believe the circumstance is affecting you even when you can't change the situation. For example, to can change your unhappiness thought with some thoughts that bring you joy or happiness.

You can change the way you respond

If you respond to things right away without giving a thought, you may not be able to manage your feelings. You need to regulate your emotions so that you can get control of your response too. For example, when you feel angry or anxious because of something, you should close your eyes and cool yourself down. In that way, you will not have to do anything stupid or be rude to someone. Similarly, if you find that you can't stop laughing in a situation where another person is sad or not smiling, try to force yourself to stop. You might not be able to change your mood but change your facial expression.

You become responsible to the way you think

You are responsible for what you feel when someone makes you angry and how you respond to your emotions. No one can make you feel the way they want if you don't allow them. You can decide to view things in another perceptive such that you will not let them make you angry. You might be expecting someone; they are late, and, in your perception, you don't think its right, but to them, it is no big deal. In that case, you should take responsibility for your emotions and try to view things positively. Note that people behave in a certain way because of different things such as beliefs, life experiences, culture, and upbringing. That means they can make you angry or happy without them knowing, and it's your responsibility to know how to respond to their actions.

What is Emotional Intelligence?

Emotional intelligence can be defined as the ability to know and control your emotions and emotions of the people around you. It is also the ability to control the feelings and use then in your thinking and solving your problems. There are several ways to increase your EQ:

You can improve emotional intelligence by using an assertive form of communication. When you use assertive communication, you give out your opinion with respect, and others no can annoy you.

You need to respond to conflict instead of reacting. When you are in dispute, a feeling of anger will arise, and you need to stay calm about it. You improve the emotional intelligence when you don't react but control your anger.

Make sure that you use active listening skills when you are in a conversation with another person. You improve your emotional intelligence when you listen carefully and understand before you respond. In that way, there will be no misunderstanding, and it shows that you have respect for the other person.

You also increase your emotional intelligence when you stay motivated at all times. You should be self-motivated and have an attitude that excites you. In that way, you will not have to deal with feelings such as sadness and disappointments.

You can also improve emotional intelligence by having positive attitudes. A negative attitude is dangerous, and you can even infect others. In that case, ensure that you have a way of having a positive attitude every day. Do things that make you optimistic.

You improve your emotional intelligence by practicing self-awareness. It is best to be aware of your emotions and how they can affect the people that are around you.

Be friendly and approachable too. That means that you need to use the right social skills according to the relationship you have with those around you. Show a positive presence such that people can approach you when they a problem.

You can also improve your emotional intelligence by empathizing with other people. Showing empathy is a sign of emotional strength and not a weakness.

How You Can Benefit From Emotional Intelligence

Emotional intelligence can benefit you in the following aspects:

- Emotional intelligence can be applied when you are in an argument or a conversation with the other person. It helps you to listen carefully before giving your response.

- You can use emotional intelligence when you are angry, and instead of expressing your feelings to others, you calm yourself down.
- You can also use emotional intelligence when you conflict. It will help you respond to it instead of reacting.
- When you have problems instead of overthinking, you use emotional intelligence to solve your problems.
- You can apply it when you make a mistake and accept you did it and apologize
- Having emotional intelligence can help you to forget a lousy moment easily and be able to move on.
- You can use emotional intelligence to get along with different people and situations
- It can be applied to change criticism to a constructive one without blaming the other people.

Short List of Ways to Help with Overthinking

Which keeps people apart from the real life they really want to continue living?

We'd all agree that such viral and damaging aspect is that they really don't know how to prevent overthinking. Here are some ways to help someone who overthinks:

- Bring matters into a broader context.
- Establish short decision timescales.
- Stop pushing the morning up for anxiety and overthinking.
- Be an Action Person.
- Remember you can't manage anything.
- Tell stop in a position you know you can't think clearly
- Do not lose out in abstract doubts.

- Make it through.
- Get more than enough healthy sleep.
- Be mindful or the present.

CHAPTER 11:

Stop Overthinking about the Past and Future

Why Do We Overthink the Past?

Each one of us has felt regret in the past. You may have gotten over them by now, but you have undoubtedly experienced how heavy regrets can be.

Regret can be something you have done—whether deliberately or unintentionally—that have hurt yourself or somebody else. You may also feel regret after making a snap decision that resulted in something less favorable than it should have been had you only taken your time.

Having regrets is a typical human experience. Obsessing over them, however, is not healthy nor productive, and would most likely result to overthinking which in turn would produce bouts of anxiety, negative thoughts and worry. There is no way to go back in time and change the circumstances that have led to those regrets. The only way to go is forward.

Why We Should Let Go of the Past

To overcome a regretful mindset, you must learn how to adapt and apply gratitude in your life. Rather than ruminating about what has happened and what could have been, you should switch your attention to the good things that are happening in your life.

Changing the way, you think is not something you can do half-heartedly. You must learn how to practice gratitude whichever way you can. You can do it by literally keeping track of the fortunate instances you have experienced in life. Others find the habit of writing down positive things to help keep them grateful, especially during tough times.

You can even take this further by being thankful for the lessons you have gained from your past, no matter how painful or hard they are. Be grateful that you have managed to live through them, and you have then been given the opportunity to learn from your past mistakes. You are now a step closer to enlightenment and becoming a better version of you.

Take note that successfully overcoming your regrets does not happen overnight. You must be patient with yourself, and continually practice applying gratitude in all aspects of your life. The more you practice it, the easier it becomes to access a grateful mindset, even during trying times.

Why We Should Not Project Negative Thinking into Our Future

Living in the present can be a difficult feat to achieve for many. Whether it is through their upbringing or as a result of various environmental factors, most people have been conditioned to dwell about the past and to worry about the future. Even today's technology contributes to one's inability to focus on the present.

Take, for example, the notifications you receive from your phone. You may be fully engrossed in whatever you are doing at the moment. Still, when you hear your phone go off, the mind tends to automatically switch to either a past experience or a future event related to the notification you have received.

Feeding negative thoughts will cause the two factors:

- The natural tendency of the mind to edit out the positive aspects of your past experiences, thus making the past seem more negative than it was; and
- The uncertainty of the current situation you are in, which then generates feelings of anxiety, negative thoughts, and worry.

Many people find it challenging to overcome these elements and start living in the present. Some do not even know what it means to be in the present. They cannot imagine how it feels like to be free from their ruminations about the past, and their apprehensions about the future. Most of the time, they simply do not have enough personal will to focus on what is currently happening to them.

Fortunately, there are various ways to get over the challenges of being in the here and now. Through the right mindset and a positive attitude, you can start living in the present and make better life choices.

How to Minimize Risks by Planning the Future

When you live in acceptance of what has already happened, and what will come to pass, then you will begin seeing things for what they indeed are. You will be able to forgive yourself and others for the mistakes that have been made in the past. You will also be able to free yourself from feelings of anxiety and worry about the things that may come your way.

Let me share my personal experience on this subject!

So, it just happens that I had made at some point in my life, quite too many financial mistakes and bad financial investments that did cost me some huge chunk of my savings for the supposed pleasant life I looked forward to living. Not once, not twice, not even thrice. Under these circumstances, I should have typically read the signs on the wall, right? And know what investment is good and bad, but duh! I kept sinking in much money in more investments, but this time around, in a bid to recover my past financial losses. However, I ended up losing more and more. At a point, I lost it and went into bouts of anxiety, negative thoughts, and worries about the mess I created in my finances and how I should have known better after the initial three losses incurred. I would overthink what would become of my financial status, especially at the point of my life where I was somewhat out of a job. I was scared, unhappy, and angry every other day I lived. This feeling went on for as long as I could remember, and then, on one Tuesday morning, I laid woken right on my bed and looked up, gazing into the ceiling before me, and I asked myself, a life-changing question.

"How has my overthinking of the past financial mistakes, what I could have done differently, and what the life I hoped to live in the future has helped me achieve?"

I decided that I was going to leave the past mistakes where it belongs, "the past"— I was going to focus on living in the present by making the most out of it— and that I wasn't going to beat myself up about what the future holds. Consciously deciding on this gave me a great sense of relief and peace.

No matter how much we try, we can't change the past merely because it is out of our control, and no matter how we wish we could predict the future, we simply can't because the universe operates on its terms and conditions. So then, the obvious choice you can make, one which you have control of is to live in the moment and enjoy what each day brings. It sure helps.

How to Use the Resources You Have with a Positive Approach

Torturing yourself with the question "what if" gives you nothing but unnecessary feelings of anxiety, negative thoughts, and worry. There is no way to know for sure what will exactly happen by choosing to act in a certain way. It is a waste of time and energy to think about the uncontrollable aspects of the future.

More often than not, obsessing over the possible outcomes of your actions will only make you feel upset. Having no definite answer since there is an endless number of possibilities can be particularly unsettling.

To stop asking yourself this question, you must:

- focus on the here and now of the situation;
- identify the things that are within your control; and
- think of each case as an opportunity to learn.

If you do end up acting upon the wrong decision, the only healthy thing to do is to learn from it and move on. Do not let your mistake define your present and what your future would become.

Reallocate the time and energy you would have used in overthinking about the what-ifs of the situation into something more productive. Use that as a motivation to make better decisions the next time you are facing a similar circumstance. Remember, you can take more control over your thoughts and actions if you would simply believe you can do so.

You are in control, and you can choose how you are going to approach essential matters in your life.

From here, you can start nurturing a positive mindset that is centered on your personal growth and development. You can reframe your outlook in life, thus giving you hope and motivation to overcome the challenges that may come your way.

It should be noted that you should actively work on embracing positivity. Once you have acknowledged that you have the right to be happy and that you are ultimately responsible for your happiness, you may then proceed to apply this positive mindset in your day to day life, and the achievement of your goals.

Once you have chosen to adopt a grateful mindset fully, then you will be able to:

- feel contentment about the blessings in your life;
- gain an optimistic point of view;
- better appreciate the people around you;
- find ways to help those in need; and
- have a higher level of self-awareness.

Accepting Life Changes Gracefully

You need to make the most out of the life you currently have by finding happiness, purpose, and satisfaction in your life.

A lot of people tend to forget that they have a choice on how to live their lives. They let themselves be stuck in their miserable situations, complaining and whining about how unfair everything is around them.

It is natural for humans to dream for the best possible future for them. However, this can only go so far if that is the only thing that you will do. You have to accept these changes and live your life in the best possible way. This goes beyond simple wishful thinking. It involves finding your real purpose in life and pursuing your passions.

Living up to your full potential is only one way to go about this, though. You can also aim to live a well-balanced life. By figuring out the right balance in the critical areas of your life, you would be able to go after the things that will make you happy and fulfilled.

To live your best life, you must commit to creating this kind of life for yourself. You have to commit to facing the challenges of personal growth and development. Only then can you have the strength, courage, and determination to live your best life.

How to Identify Things You Would Like to Achieve in the Future

Where else would you would rather be in 3 years, 8 years, or even in the next year? Such areas become your goals and while you may realize you would not want to remain still in that position as you may be now, it isn't always easy to define whatever your ultimate objectives are.

Below is a guide on how to plan for your goals for the future:

- Generate a checklist of the planned goals.
- Assume the time span for accomplishing the objective
- Start writing the priorities down clearly
- Write down what you need to do with any single goal
- Set down the Time span with clear and measurable date and time
- Timing your To-Dos
- Evaluate Development

CHAPTER 12:

Solutions to Different Topics You May be Overthinking

Stop Overthinking about the Fears of Getting Sick

A ll of us experience this anxiety, the fear of getting sick. Sometimes, we get paranoid with just a cough because we think it may lead to something serious.

Our parents play a significant role in why we get this anxiety over getting sick. From the time we were born, our parents made sure we would live a comfortable and healthy life. Some parents have influenced us that getting sick should never happen.

In addition, the social media world has taken control of almost every part of our daily lives. Studies indicate that the more hours you waste on social media platforms, the more prone you are to grow depression and experience different fears including getting sick. Consequently, it is advisable to cut out the use of social media to lessen anxiety and psychological disorder. Put off your telephone and computer for several hours each day to develop your frame of mind and reconnect with the people around you.

It is essential to have a positive mindset in life. Our well-being depends on how strong we believe that we are healthy inside and out. Taking time off to relax might be useful for your frame of mind, psychological physical condition, and sense of worth. Practice at least a single thing each day that makes you feel excellent. Listen to good songs, study the latest skill, take a long shower, or create a pleasant meal.

Stop Overthinking in Bed

When we go to bed at night, hundreds of questions and thoughts come into our mind. This is because your brain is less distracted during the night. This is the time that you relax and your mind is calmer. During the day, we tend to get very busy that our brains just brush off the thoughts we have deep inside.

Moreover, that is a healthier tone to set that signifies a sense of self-importance and achievement. Taking control and completing easy tasks shall offer you the basis to take on more during the day.

Meditate

Including some sort of mindfulness practice such as meditation into your day-by-day morning schedule might assist ground you and prepare your mind and sentiments, which then sways how you respond to challenges during your day.

Exercise

Whether it is a natural yoga schedule or a fast stroll with your pet or a speedy set of sit-ups; starting the day with movement strengthens the body and the brain. Decide what type of exercise is correct for you and program it. It does not have to be complicated, extensive, or extreme, but having some, kind of physical movement in the morning shall make your blood moving and assist quiet any psychological chatter. You may switch up what type of exercise you do each day to keep your schedule appealing.

Bathe

Taking a shower has a method of shocking your coordination and getting your transmission going. If you completely cannot get yourself into the washroom, then at a minimum do a regular washing of your face and end with a splash of freezing water. You will appear and feel more conscious than you could if you could simply walk out of bed.

Stop Overthinking about Others Judgment

Human as we are, the opinion of others always makes a significant impact on us. From the way we look to the way we dress, we are all afraid to be judged. We tend to be very conscious about the way we're living because we're so scared of what other people would say.

There are many things you can do to stop this unhealthy habit. Here are some:

Practice Gratefulness

Before you move out of bed, offer yourself a couple of minutes to smile and put into practice gratefulness. When you smile, it notifies your brain to discharge the feel-fine neurotransmitters. The released element boosts your humor, calm down your body, and lowers your heartbeat. Who could not desire to begin their day on this encouraging note?

As you smile, begin to reflect on the issues that you are thankful for before moving to the next subject. Studies have revealed practicing gratefulness lessens anxiety hormones and boosts mood. Consequently, adding a straightforward daily gratefulness practice is an enormous way to begin your day.

Start by taking a single minute in bed before you wake up to reflect on an individual and an occasion you are thankful for in your life.

Eat a Well-Balanced Breakfast

You have noted that breakfast is the most significant dish of the day. When you take time to consume a substantial breakfast, you shall have more liveliness during the day and a stronger aptitude to concentrate and focus.

Do What You Adore

If your enthusiasm is playing football, writing poetry, or showing kids how to swim, take time to do it. You shall discover that when you are doing what you adore, you are occupied with happiness.

Stop Overthinking about Losing your Friends or Partner

The fear of getting abandoned by our friends or our partner haunts us every day. Acceptance is the most significant key to stop this fear. In life, losing someone happens whether you like it or not. It is entirely unavoidable. So we should cherish every single moment that we have with them and make sure that we show them our love and kindness.

Other solutions to stop this habit are:

Assist Others

Occasionally after we have accomplished our personal objectives, we still feel unaccomplished inside since we have not made a significant contribution to somebody else's life. When we help others, it sounds excellent to be of service to somebody else. The contribution we make seems fulfilling and is a huge potential basis for our cheerfulness.

Spend Your Time with Other People

When you share your feelings, your time, and your skills with others you feel suitable for it. Time spend without sharing may be lonely. When you spend time with other people, they will feel good towards you and assist you to have more happiness in your life.

Look for a Life Instructor

A life trainer shall assist you to assess your life and why you are not feeling joyful. Maybe have limiting thinking or you have a sentimental obstruct without understanding. By taking to a life teacher, you might discover why you are dejected and what you might do to feel good.

Learn to Forgive

Keeping a grudge shall hurt you more than the other individual. You should take notice of how you think when you release your rage. Concentrate on a good future and you shall feel good.

Stop Overthinking about Finding Making it Wrong

Our mistakes don't define us. They are part of what and who we've become. All those scars we have are the proofs that we have strived hard and survived this problematic like. You will not grow without those mistakes. We should be thankful for those trials because it made us become a stronger and better person today.

Some other tips to stop this habit are:

Take a Stroll in Nature

Walking in nature might be uplifting and renewing, mainly when you are living in an artificial world. Strolling in your neighborhood park and getting fresh air might let you understand the attractiveness of the natural world.

Generate a Daybreak Habit to Focus Your Brain

Perhaps the most significant constituent of a busy morning is your schedule. Almost every productivity specialist suggests a morning schedule, though each one is just a bit diverse.

Ideally, not every daybreak habit works for everyone; however, there are fundamentals that make the morning schedule most valuable. If you examine productivity specialists' morning schedule, you will discover a few components in common. They have a constituent of focus on big picture goals, gratefulness, and arranging for the days' time.

Read Books

Reading books is a useful technique for gaining knowledge and arouse inventiveness. Fascination reading develops concentration and has a soothing effect related to meditation. Additionally, reading prior to sleeping might assist you in sleeping well. True-life books are an outstanding instrument to widen the horizon, build up new ideas, and search for motivation. Additionally, they present actionable guidance on how to conquer all sorts of challenging circumstances through real-life instances.

Appreciate

It is easy to be trapped up in the rat contest and overlook how lucky you are. Practicing appreciation is an excellent technique to generate positivity, lessen stress, and boost your physical wellbeing. How can you nurture this healthy routine? Institute a gratitude diary, volunteer, take time to value your treasured ones and tell yourself of at least a single subject you are thankful for each day before going to sleep. The more you value the small happiness of life, the better you will feel.

Stop Overthinking about Money

No matter how much money you've got, how young you're, and how big you owe, money's a problem. A new year will be an ideal time not just to improve the wealth, as well as to improve the relationship with cold cash and avoid those conscious thoughts from winning control.

Money is just a tool that gives us a feeling of security. Often times, we are too caught up in thinking of ways on how to earn more money that we are slowly disconnecting from reality.

Panicking can't get you anywhere. Your financial condition will remain the same even if you stay around feeling bad during the day or not.

Your credit score does not increase unexpectedly, since it feels bad towards you. Not just that, getting blinded by this kind of pessimism implies you have much less time to reflect as well as concentrate on much more meaningful activities.

Some tips to overcome this habit are:

- Actually live
- Speak up your worries Plan a strategy
- Fully understand your figures

Understand how much you require, and exactly what you want to do. Place a number on it, and understand what you ask. Otherwise the unclear demands would yield unclear outcomes.

Stop Overthinking about Finding Someone to Love

It's not really exciting to see your buddies form a relationship when you're still alone. Why then is your romantic happiness still not coming on through? I don't really have a reply to this one, but I'm going to tell you that there's really no excuse to bother running between attempting to find "the one." Go forward with and shake your head, because when it starts to happen, it should actually occur.

Loneliness is a feeling you get from being single. We imagine a lot of things in our mind. The things we would do if we ever found our other half. So while we're still waiting, we shouldn't feel lonely. There are a lot of different things that we can do and enjoy while patently waiting.

Some reasons why we should to stop this habit are:

- You'll feel stressed out
- This only drives others out
- And besides desperation is not attractive
- You are going to attempt to pressure yourself to like somebody
- Love needs some time
- It is indeed beautiful to be single
- Love has no deadline
- Life has much more to give than dating a guy
- You may miss the real person
- It merely adds to worse relationships
- You may never understand exactly what loving is

CHAPTER 13:

Reprogramming Your Thoughts

Why Anxious Thoughts Grow When Avoided

Stress and pessimistic mentalities go together. The nervous ideas are probably embedded in anxious emotions which have never been upheld all along way, but if those dark thoughts go uncontrolled, those who result in negative sentiments which contribute to disastrous emotions Such bad feelings are omnipresent and contagious; they have such a way of distributing to any and all kinds of many feelings, gradually manipulating your entire behavior patterns until you're mostly speaking in negativity instead of optimistic, that can be harmful to the whole career. People try to avoid anyone whose thoughts become embedded in pessimism — individuals don't like to get themselves contaminated. Others who are pessimistic are hard to accept, mainly since most people appear to be focused with self-improvement. Thus, those of us who are cynical are also overwhelmingly ignored by everyone around them that even further amplifies the anxious feelings.

The easiest way of doing this is to indulge in self-reflection or guided imagery, when you're about to recognize your negative feelings. People are actually sorting over their emotions as you're doing it, seeking to comprehend whatever the origin of the doubts that you have are. Once you're at the center of a cycle of thinking you recognize the negative feeling you've had. The pessimistic source is accountable for all that comes after it, so you should start addressing that source explicitly if you understand what it really is, and making it a case for clearing it. While you participate in this phase, you must basically ask yourself again and again how or why it means to you, based on what provides the most significance within this given circumstance.

Controlling Your Thoughts with Journaling, Reflection and Meditation

For most people, half the time we spend awake, we spend thinking or worrying about something. We're not focused on the present, and we're not actively thinking about what we do. We either go through the motions automatically, or we rush through without paying attention. We're only not paying attention enough. As it turns out, approximately 50% of the time, these participants found that their minds were not focused on their current task. Moreover, the participants realized that wandering minds led to higher levels of unhappiness since they were not focused on the task at hand.

Meditating - You'll notice that this method is encouraged a lot when you're trying to overcome your anxiety. But this is by far one of the best ways out there that gives your mind the training it needs to learn how to focus on the present. Meditation is not always about sitting in silence and trying not to think about anything as you will yourself to relax. On the contrary, meditation is linked to a myriad of psychological and neurological benefits. By being mindful and deliberately slowing down our thoughts, we're quieting the areas in the brain that is responsible for all that unnecessary noise and chatter. Trying to sit in silence and not let your scattered thoughts take center stage is going to be hard at first, but it gets easier with practice. All you need to do is find something to focus on, and in meditation, that focus can be your breath or a mantra that you repeat. Each time your mind starts to wander (and it will), don't get stressed about it. Stay calm, and simply return to focusing on your breath or mantra. That's what practice is all about.

Journaling and Talking- Anytime you feel you need a shoulder to cry on, talk to someone. Being stuck in your negative thoughts is not always easy to overcome alone is learning to recognize when you need help. Talking about your problems can be therapeutic. It gives you some release, a way to channel the emotions that you've been keeping locked away inside. If you've ever tried this method before, do you notice how much better it feels to get something off your chest? Not to mention how having someone to talk to can put things in a different perspective and shed a different light on a situation. The very act of talking about it can turn your incoherent thoughts around so you, in turn, can understand them better. Not only is this a tool in helping you overcome the mindset that has been holding you back all this time but seeing your thoughts in a different way enables you to develop a new relationship with them too. Perhaps instead of seeing them as the enemy, these thoughts can now be viewed as the very thing needed to encourage you to make a change for the better.

Reflection- Reflection is an effective way for you to be able to control your own thoughts. The demanding and hectic pace of today's lifestyle has led to the false belief that you're increasing your productivity when you multitask. Nothing could be further from the truth. Our minds were only made to focus on one thing, one stimulus at a time. Thus, it is essential to reflect on what we have done at then of the day.

Excuses are for someone who lacks discipline, and if you're serious about overcoming your anxiety once and for all, it's time to leave the excuses at the door where they belong. Holding on to your excuses only gives you a reason to continue to worry, fret, and indulge in the negative behavior patterns that are not helping you in any way. Discipline means staying focused on what you need to do and pushing aside everything else that threatens to distract you.

Recognize Thoughts as a Product of the Brain

Our brains are the ones producing the thoughts we think and have every day. These perceptions or beliefs that you hold about yourself will determine your mental attitude, the outlook you have about life in general, the way you approach the situations you're faced with and determine the behavior you exhibit in response to what you're going through. When you believe you can achieve something and you accomplish it, you have the right mindset to make it happen.

The subconscious mind is a mix of repetition and emotion, but the thing is, you need to feed your mind with statements it can accept. That's how you get it to change.

Visualization is an exercise that helps you focus your mind on the positive outcomes that you want to achieve. Seeing these happy images in your mind keeps you focused and motivated to do something about it, so they don't remain just visions in your mind. The idea behind visualization is that your mind is powerful enough to conjure up any image that you want. Anything is possible if you can think about it and picture it clearly.

Ways of Changing Your Mindset

Your mind will determine your success. What you think you will become. Believe you're going nowhere in life, and that's precisely what will happen. Believe that you're destined for success, and success will find its way to you. We often underestimate how powerful the inner monologue of the mind can be. But think about this for a moment. If you can envision all the catastrophic outcomes with clarity - and on the rare occasion it does happen, you think, "See! I knew this would happen!" - Then you can do the opposite too. The Growth Mindset is the driving force that people rarely ever talk about. It can drive you to success, or it can drive you to failure. The difference is going to boil down to which mindset you allow yourself to hold onto.

The Growth Mindset

Growth Mindset is the one you want to work on developing. This mindset is the one that lets you embrace the failures and setbacks you experience, seeing them as lessons to be learned from. This is the mindset that allows you to critically analyze, change, and adapt your behavior to suit the situation. This is the mindset that will strongly influence the kind of success you achieve throughout your life. Individuals with the Growth Mindset stand firm on the notion that effort matters most, and they are willing to learn, adapt, grow, and do whatever it takes to get what they want. They are resilient and bold, never backing down in the face of a challenge. That's the kind of mindset you need to strive for now as you work to overcome your anxiety. This notion forms the core of their belief system. To these individuals, talent and brains are only the beginning.

As soon as you change your mindset, your behavior will start to change too. To supercharge your development of the Growth Mindset, these are the other mindsets that need to exist too:

The Trust Mindset - Trust in yourself. You need to believe in your capabilities because no one else can do it for you. If you don't trust that you have it in you to do what it takes to succeed, then nothing is ever going to change. That trust in yourself needs to be so strong that it can overcome the negative inner monologue that wants to be in control. Never give up on yourself; you have more to give than you think you do.

The Patience Mindset - There's a fine line that separates standing still and moving forward in life. Being patient doesn't mean you remain stagnant. It means you wait until the most opportune moment to make your move when the time is right.

The Courage Mindset - Dealing with anxiety means you spend most of your time being afraid. Fear may be part of being human, but so is courage. After all, the fight in the fight or flight response implies that it takes courage to stand up and face your fears. You've got both these response possibilities within you, which means you're just as capable of both. It's now a matter of developing that courageous mindset, so that is the one that wins at the end of the day. Like the muscles in your body, courage is something that needs to be exercised to grow more robust, and it is one of the reasons they encourage those struggling to overcome their anxieties to face their fears instead of running from them.

The Learner's Mindset - Almost every experience in life is a lesson, even the defeats that you go through. Remember that the Growth Mindset always views circumstances and situations as a lesson to be learned from. In every setback, there is a lesson waiting to be learned. If you can cultivate the learner's mindset, that's when real growth can begin to happen. If you're willing and determined to keep learning, nothing can stand in your way. Not even the negative inner monologue.

CHAPTER 14:

Neuroplasticity

The Brain's Ability to Reorganize Itself

When living with anxiety, it is easy to become nervous over the new and unexpected. There are numerous times where we find ourselves jumping in and assuming that we are going to live our lives by strictly following a particular philosophy. This simply creates anxiety when it comes to living your life. Scientific studies have taken strides to provide that you can rewire your brain and ultimately change how it works. This will help you understand how it is possible to rewire your mind through a process called neuroplasticity. Through this process, you can overcome anxiety and as a result, prevent yourself from overthinking.

Neuroplasticity refers to the ability of the brain to restructure itself by developing new neural connections throughout life. It is through this restructuring of the mind that new nerve cells are designed to compensate for disease or injuries that one might have suffered. The nerve cells then adjust accordingly to environmental changes and new situations.

In simpler terms, neuroplasticity refers to the plasticity of your brain. This refers to the ability of your mind to change and adapt as you go about life. Depending on your environment, your brain activity will determine this change.

Examples of Neuroplasticity

Neuroplasticity, which is the capacity of the mind to adapt in reaction towards its surroundings and also to continue to evolve. Changes may occur rapidly or gradually, and could be either favorable or unfavorable.

Some of the examples of neuroplasticity are:

- Getting better from neurological damage
- ADD, ADHD, Brain Plasticity and OCD
- Improving Intellectual Efficiency

How do I Rewire My Brain from Anxiety?

There is an interesting way in which neuroplasticity helps us to understand how our minds react when we are anxious. There is a connection between the brain's flight and fight response in relation to anxiety triggers. This connection is created by neuroplasticity for anxiety. Each time you feel anxious, the mind bolsters the connection which makes you more anxious. Take for example a situation where you are involved in a car accident. In this regard, the brain will develop a connection between cars and the panic you experienced.

Luckily, there is a way of overcoming such connections of anxiety through neuroplasticity. This process works by removing the connections that you once had, thereby eliminating your anxiety.

There are numerous benefits of neuroplasticity. The primary importance of this process in this case is that it is a natural remedy to cure anxiety. Other benefits of neuroplasticity are listed below.

- Changes your habits

- Reduces stress

- Eliminates brain connections between our fears and fear triggers

- Rewires your brain to reduce anxiety

- Enhances your mind's sense of optimism

- Alters how anxiety affects you

The brain's plasticity will not be affected positively when your mind is thinking negatively. The brain will find it difficult to adjust to any changes that it might require. As a result, it is vital that you develop a positive mindset for optimal functioning of the brain's plasticity.

It's no secret that achieving a positive mindset is not easy. After all, we are all inclined to think negatively due to negativity bias. This is the main reason why it is essential to remind yourself of the significance of thinking positively always. Fortunately, this can be achieved through the use of affirmations and positive mantras.

The Happy Hormones (DOSE)

Dopamine

Dopamine encourages you to act quickly towards your aspirations and provides people the pleasure-enhancing rise once you achieve them. Anxiety, self-doubt, and lack of motivation are all related to low dopamine rates. Research show anyone with reduced dopamine levels have often gone for just a more straightforward choice and those with more substantial hormone levels have made every effort to get twice the benefit.

Split broad objectives up into tiny pieces. Instead of only encouraging the mind to rejoice whenever you cross the large end point, you should build a couple of specific mile markers for regular release of dopamine.

It's necessary to effectively rejoice — buy alcohol, or go to your local bar anytime you achieve a small target.

Serotonin

Whenever you become substantial or relevant, serotonin streams out. There is isolation and sadness because there's no serotonin. This is why people would fall towards gangs and illicit behavior — cultural norms and 'group' promote the production of serotonin. Bad lifestyles that search for help are a plea for much of what serotonin offers.

It helps the mind to recreate the past by focusing on the past accomplishments. The mind gets difficulty differentiating between what's real and what's perceived and that in many instances it releases serotonin. With this cause, activities of appreciation are prevalent; these are representations and mental images of all positive work you've done. When during a stressful day you could use a serotonin recharge take a minute or two to focus on some of your past successes and accomplishments.

Oxytocin

Oxytocin release builds trust, motivation and enhances connections. It is produced upon orgasm by males and females, also during labor and breast-feeding by moms. Animals will be rejecting their young if oxytocin production is hindered. Oxytocin improves faithfulness; men in romantic relationships provided a dose of oxytocin engaged with young women at a higher physical pace versus people who did not receive oxytocin at all. Oxytocin is the adhesive which ties loving relationships around.

Sometimes known to as the "hug hormone," giving anybody a hug is an effective way to keep the oxytocin circulating. Not only does the physical interaction increase oxytocin but this also decreases heart stress and strengthens the immune system.

Endorphins

Release of endorphins mostly as remedy to anxiety and suffering, and may reduce stress. A roaring "speed burst" and the melancholic "fast athletes" originate from endorphins while racing. Linked to morphine, it serves as local anesthetic and diminishes the sense of failure.

Laughing has been one of the simplest things to create endorphin production, as well as exercising. Also, laugher's excitement and enthusiasm, e.g. to watch a sitcom, raises endorphin rates. Bringing your sense of fun to function, sending out the humorous message and having a few moments to chuckle about throughout the day are perfect ways of keeping the endorphins streaming.

Mindful Meditation and CBT

The concept of neuroplasticity might appear daunting at first. Surprisingly, it's quite easy to manipulate. The only thing that you need is to develop specific neuroplasticity techniques aimed at helping the brain to change its brain activity.

Meditating daily can have a significant impact on your life. Based on the neuroplasticity process, meditation enhances the brain's gray matter. This is achieved by utilizing your brain's neuroplasticity potential. Regular meditation can alter the sensory perceptions that you might have developed over the years. Therefore, instead of having a negative perspective towards life, you develop a more positive attitude.

Put merely, binaural beats is a form of Cognitive Behavioral Therapy. In this form of therapy, one is required to listen to two different sound frequencies played at the same time. The frequency of the left ear will be different to the frequency of the right ear, but the mind perceives the sound as one. For instance, if the right ear notes a tone at 250 Hz and the left ear notes a tone at 240 Hz, it means that the binaural beat heard is -10 Hz. This is the difference between the two frequencies. Experts who advocate for binaural beats argue that the therapy has a similar effect to that of meditation. Potential benefits of binaural beats are as follows:

- Reduced anxiety

- Increased concentration

- Increased confidence

- Increased motivation

- Deeper meditation

- Reduced stress

Just like meditation, when using binaural beats, it is imperative that you find a suitable time where you are not interrupted. Therefore, this is an exercise that you can't combine with other tasks. You should listen to binaural beats for about 15-30 minutes in a quiet place. More importantly, you should be patient without expecting immediate results after listening to the audio for a few days. Make it a habit to spare about 30 minutes to listen to binaural beats for a month or two. This is an excellent way in which you will experience the potential benefits listed above.

Mindfulness is yet another technique that will help you tap into your brain's plasticity. This is because mindfulness has a positive impact on helping rewire the brain to think positively. Consequently, by living mindfully, one can reduce stress and increase their sense of optimism towards life. In addition, living mindfully also reduces anxiety as it advocates for the idea of living in the moment.

Find a Strong Purpose

Neuroplasticity is a complex concept that you might not have heard of before. However, the process reiterates some .of the things that we have talked about in this guide. The point of neuroplasticity is that it depicts how the brain changes its activity.

Under circumstances, you should find a strong purpose inside your brain. This help you process positive thoughts in the past that would help you deal with the present situation. It can be said that it's the brain's way of adapting to your life's changes. Neuroplasticity can be used to remedy anxiety because it removes any existing connection that you have between anxiety and anxiety triggers. Accordingly, it prevents you from being in panic mode whilst driving a car because you once had a car accident.

CHAPTER 15:

Behavioral Neuroscience

Why Behavioral Neuroscience is Important?

Behavioral Neuroscience, also called Behavioral Analysis, explores the interrelationship in between mind, the environment, and the living things' behavior.

Behavioral science published studies provide us with the solutions to identify a range of issues that the world is facing by expanding our opportunity to measure, comprehend, anticipate, enhance, and regulate people's behavior. Work by Behavioral psychologists has developed our understanding of a variety of issues, include but are not confined to dependency neuroscience, ageing, fatigue, anxiety, depression, autistic disorder, schizophrenia and immune system deficiencies.

How the Brain Affects our Behavior

Your conscious and aware mind is what your friends and family would use to identify who you are. This is the result of how you live your day to day life and the reactions you display for specific situations. However, this does not mean that this is the location that controls the mind and all the actions of your body.

Your consciously aware mind is also a small portion of the brain's functions, like a ship captain who is perching on the bow of the ship spouting orders. It is the crew's primary responsibility to follow through with the orders that have been spouted to them from the captain. This is what the unconscious does for the body and mind, and the subconscious works to relay what to do. The captain is the primary person that is leading the crew on the ship and is the specific one to provide all the orders for the crew to follow. However, the crew is primarily responsible for carrying out the orders and tasks for that ship. This is an excellent metaphor for how the subconscious and conscious mind works to control the body.

The consciously aware mind is able to communicate your character and needs to surface which relays the inner voice, as well as physical actions, pictures, and writing abilities. Your mind is the control system for recollections of memories, as well as contact with the continuous unconscious resources. The mind will use your unconscious as the station that holds all recollections from past experiences. This process can be inhibited due to experiences of trauma as well as, block you from remembering things that are unfavorable to you. These memories are still accessible, just subconsciously blocked, so they do not harm you. Due to these experiences, as well as recollections you can form habits, beliefs, as well as, behaviors that are the foundation of your whole life.

The constant communication of the unconscious will take place while the awareness of the conscious mind is processing and maintaining the person's actions. This provides a connection with the intentions for every interaction that you have within the world. This will allow for a filtered habit and belief system that communicates the appropriate emotions, dreams, feelings, sensations, and imaginations.

Another common argument, made by several individuals, relates to how the mind is consciously aware of what you are doing? It can instantly connect with all of the thoughts and reasoning that is logical within your mind. However, this also does not distinguish the unconscious entirely from your subconscious. Your minds ability to be unconscious and yet store the reminiscence of the past along with the emotions, feelings, and habits and then connect them with the logic and reasoning for immediate recall, is proof in and of itself that the conscious and subconscious are always alert.

This provides the most straightforward rationalization that is found within the 2 minds. It is the most potent function which develops your consciously aware mind in order to handle the functions listed below:

1. The minds ability to focus on a specific direction.

2. The minds ability to connect the unrealistic with the imagination.

These are the 2 vital talents which will amendment your life.

The role that the subconscious mind will play in your life is magical.

Outside of your short-lived memory space, your subconscious will work in conjunction with the functioning of your daily activities. This means that it is crucial to your ability to live actively. It works arduously with certain aspects of your mind to make recollection faster and the access of your thoughts easier to process.

Things similar to the list below –

•Memories – like the experiences that you have had pastly, such as driving your car. This is something that you can consciously do without having confidence in your abilities since you have pastly learned these things. This can also include the appearance that you wish to achieve form your home's environment.

•Current activities that are a daily process for you as well as, the behaviors that you exhibit, and the mood or habits that you have.

•Filters, which pertains to beliefs as well as value systems- These are used to process the data that is checked for validity when they take place. This keeps the balance between the perception of reality and reality. Similar to the sense that you have honed over time; sight, touch, smell, hear. This helps to distinguish between the real senses so that you can filter out the ones that have been suggested to you.

Your brain works similarly as the mind; it works to deal with a reminiscence from past experience. However, there is a distinction between each of the parts. If you consider what the image of a constellation looks like you will be able to imagine the human mind. By referring to the human brain like a constellation, you can also imagine that a layer more in-depth is the unconscious mind. Then one layer deeper is the subconscious mind. This is like seeing the constellations within the solar system and then the galaxy. Although these systems of conscious thought are causally related, they are indirectly different in many aspects. They also provide influence for separate but similar things in your mind. This means that the brain would be the cellar, and the library that is underground is the wishes and reminiscences of times gone by. This also relates to the habits, that are formed and the behaviors behind those habits. The mind is the repository for all the emotions that are deep-seated within you create the programming at birth. If you wish to make modifications that are vital to your core level, then this location within the mind is the designated location for that specific process. Although it can produce some harsh and quick results.

Developed Mechanisms of Behavior in Humans and Animals

Behavioral genetics plays a significant role in wildlife conservation. Attempts to raise endangered animals in captivity strap on comprehending the habitat requirements of the organisms, breeding behavior and relationships between parent and children.

Most life forms exist in classes, and the class reflects the degree of hierarchy, by which eco physiological events happen. As such, knowing specific mechanisms depends on awareness of the processes which enable or restrict group dynamics.

Most if not all physical processes are related scientifically, thereby having symbiotic influence on social activity. The awareness of such differential impacts, which could enhance understanding of team interactions, especially in different conditions, is a driver for growth.

Different Animal Modes

Perception is the organization, recognition and comprehension of sensory stimuli to reflect and interpret the material or environment provided. Perception relies on the human brain's diverse functions, but abstractly appears mostly seamless, since this process happens beyond conscious thought.

Sensation. The sensory system senses sensory information and channels them to the body through the nervous system. The perceptual method is founded on different cell types of the sensory neuron which turn sensory perception to increased membrane capacities.

Emotions. In general, both researchers and quasi-scientists have seemed to accept that emotions are genuine, and because they are highly beneficial to society at least, and maybe to some other species. The manifestation of animal sentiments highlighted a lot of fascinating and tough questions which were committed to limit rigorous scientific study, particularly within free-ranging organisms fairly.

Common Behavioral Symptoms of Stress

Negative thinking will often lead to stress. When you constantly dwell on negative self-talk, this is what your subconscious mind will focus on. Instead of ruminating on how bad things seem to follow you, it is vital to realize that such thoughts can have a negative impact on your emotional wellbeing.

Some common behavioral symptoms of stress are the following:

- Sadness or sense of hopelessness.
- Depression and restlessness.
- Modesty, moodiness and wrath.
- The feeling of confusion
- Alienation and separation.

Arguably, stressors will always be there. For instance, getting stuck in traffic is a common thing. It only leads to stress when you handle it in a negative way. In this regard, having a pessimistic view about traffic will cause anxiety and stress. Recognizing that you have the power to control how you think should help you recognize that you can easily evade stress. So, why should you fuss about a traffic jam when you are certain that there is nothing you can do about it? To effectively deal with such a situation, you should keep your mind engaged with something else. Listen to your favorite music as you wait for traffic to open up. Alternatively, you can listen to positive affirmations to warrant that your mind doesn't slip into negative thinking.

CHAPTER 16:

Overthinking and the Risk of Mental Health Problems

How Overthinking Affects Your Mental Health

Bad Habits

W e all know that drinking and smoking are bad habits and there are many reasons for this. One of these reasons is that such habits can cause depression and anxiety in people who indulge in these things. Drugs, tobacco and alcohol tend to cause a chemical imbalance in the brain and this is how addictions develop. This dependency on such substances can cause the person to become anxious and depressed. They especially suffer a lot when they don't have access to these things and go into withdrawal. If a person is depressed, it is important to check whether they are an addict and the root cause of the addiction before trying to treat them.

Sedentary Lifestyle

A sedentary lifestyle is not usually a healthy one and can often lead to depression in a person. People who lack any physical activity in their daily life will tend to be unhealthy and gain a lot of weight. Excessive weight issues cause people to have body image issues that can make them anxious and depressed. Women in particular get depressed when they lack any regular exercise and gain weight. They fear being judged by others and being looked down on. This lifestyle causes higher release of cortisol in the brain and depression is more likely to develop.

Insomnia

Sleep is crucial for all human beings to live a healthy life. It is important to get at least 8 hours of restful sleep every night. They will get more stressed and anxious, when a person fails to get sufficient sleep. If someone has a bad sleep cycle, it can affect everything else they do as well. People who have insomnia are susceptible to developing depression. They lose interest in life and lead a very unhealthy routine. Sleeplessness takes a heavy toll on the person's mind.

High Caffeine Intake

People love drinking coffee as soon as they wake up and to work through the day. But did you know that excessive caffeine intake could lead to depression? People who consume too much tea or coffee will be prone to getting anxious and depressed. The caffeine causes the brain to process certain chemicals in a different way than it should normally. Such people will also find it hard to get sufficient sleep and this can be another factor that causes depression.

Childhood Issues

If a child undergoes a traumatic incident like physical abuse, rape or any type of harassment, they are likely to develop depression and it carries on to adulthood. Children are very impressionable and their childhood experiences tend to shape them, as they grow older. If they suffer from any such unpleasant experiences, it can leave a very negative impact on them throughout their lives. It is important to check a patient's history to determine if they have faced any such childhood issues that could have led to depression over time.

Injuries

Suffering from head injuries is another cause for mental health issues. There are certain parts of the head that are more prone to severe injuries and it can result in physical and mental side effects. When someone takes a tumble or hurts their head, you might see them develop depression and anxiety soon. It is important to get treatment and find the real cause of it.

Bad Parenting

We all assume that all parents love and support their kids no matter what. Sadly, there are children who don't receive this from their parents and they have a higher chance of developing depression. When a child sees others getting this love and support from their parents, they compare their own and can develop a sense of loneliness and depression. Even when parents have a lot of bad habits or a bad reputation, it can affect the life of the child and cause them to get depressed. However, parents are role models for all children and they learn what they see. This causes such children to repeat the same behavior they have observed from their parents and turn into unpleasant adults. They may face issues while mingling with others and be considered unpleasant thus being another cause of depression. Hence you can see how bad parenting can be a real cause of depression too.

Loneliness

It is surprising to see how many people feel lonely these days. Even when they have active social lives and spend a lot of time with people at work, they develop a sense of loneliness. If a person does not have a supportive family, good friends or even good neighbors, they start to feel lonely. It affects their state of mind and they develop depression over time. When someone goes through the same monotonous routine every single day, things get boring and this can also cause depression. A lot of millennial move around from place to place for their jobs. This move to a completely new place requires a lot of adjusting and can be very tough when there is no one friendly or familiar around. They can get depressed at this point no matter how much the new job pays too.

Peer Pressure

Peer pressure is one of the eminent social causes of depression all over the world. When it comes to the younger generation, peer pressure may actually be one of the leading causes of such conditions. Youngsters always want to fit in and do not cope well with being singled out in a negative manner. They try their best to buy the things their friends buy or do the things they do. When they fail to do so, they develop a sense of anxiety over it and even depression. Peer pressure is especially hard for the kids who undergo bullying when they are singled out. Such cases can even lead to self-harm or even suicide.

How Overthinking Affects Your Physical Health

Common headaches

If you have headaches, you are likely to think too much. Headaches tell our bodies that we need a break; this applies to our brains as well.

Moreover, you'll find that you think the same things repeatedly if you keep a close eye on your thoughts. Worriers tend to have negative looping thought systems, so in order to counter this, gradually switch over to positive thoughts instead. Concentrate on your breathing and mindfulness, and your headaches will disappear in no time.

Muscle and joint pain

Overthinking can affect you physically after becoming a part of your psyche, and until it gets addressed, it will continue to manifest itself as phantom muscle and joint pain without any medical cause. Although overthinking starts in your head, it eventually affects the parts of your body causing exhaustion and fatigue. To avoid this, exercise regularly and stretch before going to sleep. This will help you achieve a healthy body and mind. The mind and body are closely related, so much that a decline in one's condition will negatively affect the other as well.

Fatigue

Being constantly tired indicates a problem that we need to solve. Our bodies need us to pay attention to the signals that it is sending, rather than continuing to go about our day and ignore its important messages. While fatigue is normally caused by overworking oneself, overthinking can also wear you out as well. When we quit fretting about any of it, then it makes perfect sense; you'll be pushing your brain to the limit by overthinking and burning it out eventually.

How It Can Lead to Depression

Depression, which tends to occur more in women than in men, is the direct result of these lingering thoughts. The way it manifests itself can vary depending on a person's age and gender. In men, it may be seen in symptoms such as tiredness, irritability, and sometimes anger. Men tend to behave more recklessly when they are depressed, which can be seen by their abuse of drugs or alcohol. These behaviors may often be passed off as masculine, so they are less likely to recognize it as depression and are not inclined to seek help or treatment.

Women in a depressed state are more likely to appear sad and have deep feelings of worthlessness and guilt. They may be uncertain to take part in social activities or engage with others, even those who are close to them. Depression in children will also be different. Young children may refuse to go to school or show signs of separation anxiety when parents leave. Teenagers are more likely to be irritable, sulky, and often get into trouble in school. In more extreme cases, you might see signs of an eating disorder or substance abuse.

It is normal to feel low, moody or sad once in a while. But these emotions occur to some people intensely and for extended periods. The feelings can last even for years for no apparent reason. That is depression.

Depression affects all aspect of your life. Your physical health and mental health deteriorate. It can affect to how you feel about yourself and that, in turn, affects all the other aspects of your life.

Depression Symptoms

Different types of depression have different indicators. However, some standard indicators can hint depression.

If you notice that you or someone has been feeling down, sad and miserable for most of the time and the same persists for a period longer than two weeks, then that could be a sign that you or the person in question is depressed.

Some of the common symptoms of people who are depressed include:

- Behavior
- Losing interest in having a social life
- Failing to complete your required tasks. For instance, a depressed student will suddenly stop getting school work done and even fail to show up for school

- Withdrawal from friends, family, and people that you were once close to
- Having a very short concentration span
- Emotions
- Feeling Sad
- Having guilt
- Being very irritable
- Lack of confidence in what you do
- Generally being unhappy
- Being indecisive
- Feeling disappointed
- Generally being sad
- Physically
- Being tired and exhausted at all times
- Feeling sick and run down
- Having recurrent muscle pains and headaches
- Experiencing sleeping problems
- Loss of appetite
- A significant change in weight. One can either gain a lot of weight or lose a lot of weight

How It Can Lead to PTSD and Borderline Personality Disorder

Commonly, post-traumatic stress disorder (PTSD) and borderline personality disorder (BPD) can coexist. About 15% and 50% of individuals experiencing BPD may also have PTSD — a percentage significantly higher than those in the wider public.

Studies show that the most common symptoms of these two disorders is overthinking.

The PTSD and BPD signs can indeed converge. Those with PTSD can have difficulty controlling their thoughts, and thus feel deep emotions or frequent mood changes. They struggle to control their frustration too.

CHAPTER 17:

How Overthinking Causes Serious Problems in Your Life

Very High Levels of Overthinking Can Lead to Pathological Issues

I t is not uncommon for an individual to induce a small amount anxious often. Overthinking could be an utterly cheap reaction to disagreeable situations. Individuals tend to overthink if they're having a retardant at work, throughout a check, or before a giant date. Even creating a tiny low call will cause a small amount of tension. However, there's a giant distinction between feeling Anxious once you're a stressed and mental disorder.

Anxiety disorders will be thus severe that they impede the day to day functions of individuals who are suffering from them. Within the mental state profession, a mental disorder is taken into account to be a heavy mental state. The concern and worry that an individual will feel will be constant and it will be thus severe that it will be disabling. Luckily, with treatment, an individual with this condition will overcome the disorder and live a standard life.

GAD- Generalized Anxiety Disorder

GAD is that the most typical mental disorder and other people with the disorder don't seem to be invariably able to establish an explanation for their anxiety.

Just even worrying about heading through each day creates fear. Persons with GAD do not really understand when to interrupt the anxiety process and believe that it is beyond their influence, and although they generally understand that their stress is somewhat more severe than that of the circumstances warrant. All mental illnesses can be associated with an inability to handle conflict, and several individuals with GAD seek to change circumstances. Most men feel that anxiety stops negative situation from happening and they think that giving up concerns is dangerous. Individuals will also deal with specific signs, such as nausea and dizziness.

Panic Disorder

Temporary or unforeseen attacks of intense terror and apprehension characterize anxiety disorder. Such events have caused trembling, uncertainty, migraine, or difficulty in breathing. Anxiety attacks start to occur and escalate rapidly, creeping up once in every 30 minutes. However, a scare may last for hours. Panic disorders sometimes occur once horrifying experiences or prolonged stress however might also occur while not a trigger. A person experiencing a scare might misinterpret it as a dangerous disease and will create forceful changes in behavior to avoid future attacks.

While the precise causes for anxiety and panic illness are unknown, there's a propensity in homes to get anxiety attacks. However there tends to become a link towards career changes like university graduation or moving into the workforce, tying the knot or having a child. Intense stress, including a deceased family member, breakup or job loss could also cause panic disorders.

Specific Phobias

This is often an irrational concern and rejection of a specific object or scenario. The individual with a phobia can recognize a worry as irrational or intense but remains still unable control fear about the trigger's emotions. Stimulates for a fearful derangement range through common objects to events as well as pets. Studies show that all human beings have their own phobias. Sometimes, you may not know it until you deal with it in the actual setting.

This is often a concern and rejection of places, events, or things from that it should be troublesome to flee or within which facilitate wouldn't be accessible if an individual becomes at bay. Individuals typically misapprehend this condition as a phobic neurosis of open areas and also the outdoors, however it's not thus easy. An individual with a phobia disorder might have concerns about exploit home or exploitation elevators and transport.

Social Anxiety Disorder

You all understand how anxious or awkward it feels in a public setting. Perhaps when you met somebody unfamiliar and felt shaky hands while making a huge announcement, you stayed silent. Communications skills or going into such a crowd of strangers isn't necessarily appealing to all, but more often than not, only a few people can get past it.

This is often a concern of negative judgment from others in social things or of public embarrassment. The psychological mental illness involves a range of emotions, such as nervousness, an emotional worry, and fear over shame and disapproval.

Such condition can lead people to avoid large meetings and social interaction to the extent of making daily life extremely troubled. Increased levels of stress describe social anxiety after detachment from a person or position has sense of contentment or health. Detachment usually may result in signs of distress.

OCD- Obsessive-Compulsive Disorder

Like a thread locked on an old machine, OCD causes a person to focus on a given idea or impulse. Although you do not derive some feeling of gratification from conducting such repetitive behaviors, these give some fleeting escape from the anxiety produced by those anxious thoughts.

Obsessions are repetitive thoughts, images or urges which appear in your head again and again. Such things you would not want to get but you can't ignore them. Such repetitive feelings are also disturbing and irritating.

Compulsions are actions or habits that you feel obligated to carry out constantly. Compulsions are generally done in an effort to have obsessive thoughts fall silent. If you are terrified of infection, for instance, you may establish detailed routines for tidying up. The pleasure don't ever lasts even so. In reality, the intrusive thoughts typically get louder again. Yet compulsive habits and behaviors also eventually wind up generating fear itself as they have become very much more timely and challenging.

PTSD- Post-Traumatic Stress Disorder

It's natural to feel terrified, lonely, worried, and detached, after a horrific incident. Yet if the discomfort does not in itself disappear, there might be post-traumatic stress disorder (PTSD) in yourself. For just about any issue that makes you worry for your life, PTSD may grow. Many people attribute PTSD with abuse or warfare-scarred service members — and perhaps the most main symptom among males is military involvement. However any activity, or sequence of actions that overload you with feelings of despair and powerlessness and leave you deeply broken, may cause PTSD — especially when the incident feels uncertain and unpredictable.

PTSD may impact those who encounter the terrible experience directly, all who experience the incident as well as those who subsequently clean up the mess, such as rescue teams and law enforcement agencies. Whichever the source of your PTSD, you may learn how to control your emotions through care and help, reduce traumatic experiences and step beyond the anxiety.

Common Therapies for Stress and Anxiety Issues

Below are some advanced techniques to combat with stress and anxiety:

Cognitive Behavioral Therapy (CBT)

This therapy is best-preferred approach and widely adopted for the treatment of anxiety disorders. Most researches have shown that CBT is a very effective therapeutic approach for treating social anxiety disorder and panic disorder. Basically, Cognitive behavioral therapy focused on addressing the negative thought patterns and thought distortions that affect the way we perceive ourselves and the world around us. Just as suggested by its name, CBT consists of two main components

Cognitive therapy: Cognitive therapy focuses on examining how our negative thoughts make us anxious.

Behavior therapy: Behavior therapy focuses on how an individual responds to or behaves when faced with anxiety triggering situations.

CBT bases itself on the fact that the way we feel is determined by how we think and not by external events. This means that the situation you are in does not determine your feelings. How you feel is determined by how you perceive the situation you are in.

Dialectic Behavioral Therapy (DBT)

Another form of CBT is dialectic behavioral therapy (DBT). Cognitive behavioral therapy helps to recognize and alter negative ways of thought, which advocates for constructive improvements in actions.

The word "dialectical" refers to the belief that the combination of two opposing forces in counseling — recognition and improvement — yields positive benefits than only one of the two. A distinctive feature of DBT is its emphasis on acknowledging a patient's discomfort as a way to support clinicians — and incorporating the research required to alter toxic attitude.

DBT can be used to combat risk of suicide and other self-destructive ones. It demonstrates clinical skills to deal with dysfunctional habits, and to improve them. Dialectical behavioral treatment focuses on patients at high risk, and those who are difficult-to-treat. Frequently such individuals have several conditions. The original aim of DBT has been to help people experiencing suicidal tendencies and bipolar disorder.

Schema Therapy (ST)

Schema therapy is a modern form of treatment incorporating, among others, components of cognitive behavioral therapy (CBT), psychotherapy, attachment theory, and emotion-focused treatment.

It is an overarching concept aimed at treating illnesses of individuality as well as other mental issues which does not quite often react to several other alternative treatments.

You'll meet with a counselor in schema therapy to discover and appreciate the schemes, also called maladaptive schemes. Schemas are dismissive habits which some individuals form if their thoughts and feelings as a kid were not fulfilled.

Schema therapy is aimed at teaching you how to guarantee that your interpersonal demands are fulfilled in a productive way which does not cause suffering.

Acceptance and Commitment Therapy (ACT)

Acceptance and Commitment Therapy (ACT) is a counselling technique that differs from conventional behavior therapy and dialectical behavior therapy.

Patients decide to stop ignoring, rejecting and having trouble with their thoughts and feelings. They accept instead that such broader emotions are adequate reactions to such circumstances which should not discourage them from relocating further in their daily life. With such awareness, patients start to realize their problems and sufferings and dedicate themselves to making sensible behavior changes, regardless of the outcome in their daily life as well as how they believe about all this.

The Super Skill of Mental Health

It really doesn't help when you are struggling from a crippling phobia, panic attacks, unrelenting worries or obsessive thoughts, what is more, important is that you don't have to live a life full of anxiety and fear. Anxiety and fear be treated. Therapy is the most effective option for your anxiety problem. The reason why anxiety therapy is the best option is that it differs from other anxiety medication in many ways. Anxiety therapy focuses on treating anxiety beyond just symptoms of the problem because it uncovers the main underlying causes of your fears and worries; and then teaches you how to overcome these worries and fears. Anxiety therapy will teach you how to relax, how to look at a situation from a different perspective and in less frightening ways and in the end, you will be able to develop skills on how to cope and solve your problems.

Anxiety has no fast solution. You can only be able to overcome an anxiety disorder when you take your time and be committed towards it. You are required to be ready to face your fears rather than avoiding them. Therefore, be ready to feel worse so as to get better. It is important that you stick with the treatment plan and follow the advice of your therapist. There are times that you will almost feel discouraged with your recovery pace maybe because it is taking time. I think one thing you should know is that anxiety therapy is very effective when conducted at a slower pace. Be patient, and you will see the benefits.

CHAPTER 18:

Active Problem Solving

A ctive problem solving is immediately taking on the things that worry you and then taking care of the root problem, instead of letting the ghost go and leave everything unresolved. However, active problem solving is easier said than done.

7 Problem Solving Strategies You Can Apply in Your Daily Life

Step 1 – Identify the problem

This is where you analyze your situation and then you figure out what is the root cause of all your troubles.

Step 2 – List all possible solutions

Take a seat and draw up a list among all potential ideas for fixing the issues. Take notes of what you'll do, it doesn't matter if anything seems impossible as of the moment and every concept has the capacity to affect.

When you've got that real issue, you could also have a set of alternative solutions.

Step 3 – Evaluate each option and select the best choice

Now that you have a list of the possible things that you can do, evaluate each one of them, and find out which one is the most viable course of action. Imagine what would happen if you went with a particular course of action. Will there be negative repercussions if you chose this particular plan? Toughest-case scenario: if each of your strategies seems likely to fail, which one will do you the least amount of damage?

This can be very hard to locate out which is the more feasible route to take, particularly because you may feel prejudiced toward the decisions that aren't as tough to create. In this case, it is best to run your choices to other people, like your friends, or better yet, with a lawyer so that you will know if you yourself are breaking any rules.

Stage 4- Action

When you've agreed upon a strategy, bring it into motion instantly. This isn't the moment to presume oneself second (actually don't presume oneself second because it will invoke your negative thinking illness), immediately jump into the density of it and enforce your strategy. It may seem hard yet think of that as though it was a safety pin; it would be better for you to just rip it off in one fell swoop rather than taking it slow and prolonging your agony.

During this step, ask yourself the following questions: when will you implement your plan (writing down the exact date is the best), and who will you talk to regarding this problem.

Step 5 – Does this solve your problem?

After all has been said and done, did the process solve your problem? Did you only get a partial solution, and the bulk of the problem is still there? Did things get even more complicated now? If you did not get the ideal outcome, or the result was not even worth considering as a success, go back to the third step and try again.

If you are persistent, you will most likely solve your problem, and in the event that you do, you'll have:

So, regardless if you had a lot of trouble solving the problem and it took you awhile, or if your plan went without nary a hitch and you solved the problem on your first try, you will still get a couple of bonuses once you cross the finish line.

A few of the best possible ways to handle your overthinking condition is to focus more on active problem solving rather than dwelling on the things that make you worry. When you focus on solving the problems at hand, you will not only distract yourself from the negative thoughts that came with your problems, you also prevent them from coming back to trouble you again.

Five Questions You Can Ask Yourself When Facing a Problem

1. Will it cause me regret if I don't work on this right now?

Understanding the long-term consequences of whatever choices you take seems smart, since you wouldn't want to spend eternity doing anything which you will resent in the end.

2. What causes me fear?

Persons sometimes get trapped with choices, and if they make decisions, they become afraid of what might happen.

3. Does my heart approve about what I'm feeling?

Often these gut feelings are indeed the correct ones and you'll never reach a choice which doesn't connect well in there with you.

4. To what am I actually doing this?

The sanest choices one may create are those with the goal in sight.

5. Who am I doing this for, really?

Have a realistic look at just how your decisions can help you or others in the face of a difficult life-long choice.

Tips on How to be Better at Solving Problems

Ruminating on your problems does nothing to solve them, what they do is make you feel even worse and sorry for yourself; nothing gets accomplished and the problem still remains.

On the other hand, when you take on the problem head-on, you feel empowered; you no longer feel that your life is in shambles. You start to believe that your life is manageable and not as stress-filled as you first thought it was.

Sometimes, facing problems directly is almost impossible because doing so means you will be on a head-on collision with your fears, possible conflicts, and your feelings of awkwardness. Fortunately, it does get easy over time. The amount of discomfort you will feel will gradually reduce because you know that you will no longer have a problem looming over your head once you are done solving it.

It is best that you learn this early on: active problem solving is not appropriate for all situations. Some situations are deemed unsolvable; there are some circumstances that are simply beyond your control, like the weather, how other people would react, and many others.

Take this scenario for instance: your sister is dating someone whom you do not particularly like, and you heard that the two of them are already engaged and plans on getting married soon. This decision of your sister caused you to feel anger and sadness. In this situation, you cannot apply active problem solving because you have no say on who your sister wants to marry, and the only thing that you can do now is to learn to cope using your emotion-centric skills.

Here is another scenario: you are arguing with your landlord because the heat in your apartment somehow got cut off, and you have been wearing a thick jacket indoors for three days now. In this scenario, you still need to use emotion-focused coping skills in order to get your anger back in check, but you will mostly be using active problem solving to resolve your issue with your landlord. You need to resolve this problem, or else you will be overthinking all throughout the night in a very cold apartment.

Our minds are continuously creating large bonds and improving old ones and intellectual engagement is important to aid this process. Mind games are one of the best ways not only to keep your mind intellectually engaged but also too occupied to worry and fret. So if you enjoy playing mind games, here are some of the benefits you will gain:

They are a great workout. Challenging your mind with word puzzles, logic problems and thinking games gives your brain a good workout and strengthens concentration and analytical thinking. They strengthen existing connections in the brain and forms new ones.

Better capacity to absorb and proves new information and recall memories. Puzzles and brain teasers boost both of the functions, again, by strengthening connections between neurons.

Keep your brain young and active. Brain games keep your mind active and alert to help prevent deterioration as you age.

CHAPTER 19:

Creating a Plan of Action towards Change

Action towards Change

One of the tools that you can use to deal with overthinking, anxiety, depression, and stress is creating and action towards change. This is actually a skill that people often neglect because a lot of times we tend to deal with only the emotions that affect us from day to day.

Having managing skills are necessary. They help you manage the strong emotions that you may experience. Active problem solving on the other hand is a skill that may not always address the roller coaster of emotions that you go through but it can sure help get rid of the source of your negative emotions.

Actively solving the problems that are causing you stress is a practical approach to beating overthinking and creates the change you want to achieve. You can say that it is a more lasting solution too. By dealing with the actual problems that is the root cause of your trouble, you will begin to see that life is a lot easier to manage since the stress has been reduced.

You see, if you just address the emotions and not handle the roots of those emotions then you're not getting anywhere. You will still have those triggers that cause your negative emotions. But if you actively tackle and deal with the actual problem then yes you may feel like you're still getting some kind of emotional beating but in the end, it will be the last emotional breakdown that you will ever have.

Think of it as an exchange between temporary and short-term discomfort for a longer-term solution that deals somehow solves the issue for the long term.

Changing Your Thought Patterns

Note however that not every situation can be resolved by action towards change. That means not every case of overthinking and stress related troubles can be solved by this approach. Every good thing has a limit, unfortunately. There are some situations where active problem solving just can't be applied.

Here's an example. Let's say the huge cause of your stress is the fact that you believe your sister is marrying the wrong guy. This is causing you a lot of grief and sadness. At times it may have even made you angry.

Action towards change would have had you make sure that your sister never gets married to her fiancé, but that just isn't the right thing to do now isn't it? You can't just actively solve this problem so you will just have to find another way to resolve your issues.

Let's say that the decisions and blunders of the current president of the country is causing you a lot of stress and anxiety.

What would you do about any of it? Will you start an impeachment campaign? Will you even go so far as to plan an assassination attempt? Of course not—you just can't do that and not get into further trouble and more stress and anxiety.

It will always depend on you. Your thought patterns will change depending on how well you train your mind to respond to these matters actively. If you want to change something about your emotions and feelings, you should be able to know and acknowledge first what is the reason you want to change this certain feeling about someone.

How to Write an Action Plan

Goal setting is incredibly simple but it can be challenging to develop a plan to achieve results. Even when action plans can sometimes differ significantly of assignments and timeframes, they are largely consistent with much the same framework and contain the very same data sources. Develop a plan of action to help you reach your specific goals by taking these five easy steps:

- Place Objectives and goals
- Build a check list
- Provide timetable
- Defines capabilities
- Review development

Proposed 7-Day Action Plan

Below is a systematic process that you can use to solve problems that you may encounter actively. Note that this is not the only way to apply the ideas of active problem solving. However, do take note of the details highlighted in the approach and example below.

Day 1. Identify the Problem and Its Causes

By doing so, ensure you describe definitely what problems you are trying to assess. Well, what is the problem? Be concise and try your best to be as accurate as you can at defining and identifying the actual problem.

Remember that people see a problem in different ways. Some people may not even think that there is a problem. People just have different views and that is something that you will have to deal with especially when you're trying to resolve a relationship problem.

Make sure to separate the issues that you need to deal with from the interests that are at stake while you're at it.

Day 2. Understand the interests of parties involved

Life coach and best-selling author, Stephen Covey, once explained in his book "The 7 Habits of Highly Effective People" that in order to resolve problems with other people and our relationships with others we must seek first to understand the other person and then seek to be understood that person. This is part of what Covey calls interpersonal greatness.

It is important that you understand the interests of the people involved. This is usually a critical step that is missing when people try to resolve inter personal issues – which is a pretty common thing for human beings to dabble on.

When we say "interests" we refer to the needs of the individuals involved in the issue. These are the things that need to be satisfied in order to reach a resolution. In the case of a landlord to whom you owe the month's rent, his interest is getting paid what is due to him. In the case of a child, where you missed seeing her recital, you owe emotional support.

These each interest must be enumerated and to resolve the issue you must address each one of them. There should be a list of interests and a separate list—a list of possible solutions for each interest.

Day 3. List the possible solutions

This is the part where you do a lot of brain storming. Allow plenty of room for all possible rationales. Let your creative juices to flow while you're at it.

Create a list of options. After creating that list, evaluate the potential of each option that you have on your list and strike out the ones that aren't realistic or satisfactory.

Day 4. Come up with the most feasible options

You will eventually come up with a shorter list which will contain the most feasible options. Now, analyze the pros and cons of each suggested solution. Again, take out the ones that don't have enough pros compared to the cons.

Day 5. Narrow down your list to the top 2 options

Upon having learned the advantages and disadvantages of every item on the list, narrow down your selection to the best 2 on it. Figure out if there is a way to bundle them together? If that is no possible then choose the one that has more pros than cons.

Day 6. Document everything

When a decision is made regarding the best strategic plan, then document that one too. As you write that down, think about the details of the deal that you have just made and also all of the possible implications that come with it.

Day 7. Make an agreement

Now, here's another thing that people forget to do. This works especially when dealing with relationships and other people's emotions.

Agree on the terms and conditions of the resolution or solution that works best for both of you.

It Isn't Done Yet

Now here's the thing—it doesn't mean that when you narrowed down your list of options that you automatically have found a solution that will solve the problem. Mentally weighing the options doesn't automatically make something the most beneficial solution.

Sometimes, even after selecting what seems to be the best or most logical option, and then applying it, the problem still isn't resolved. How is that possible? Here, allow me to demonstrate with an example.

Let's go back to that problem with the idle landlord. So you determined that the best course of action would be to call and write him. You called but he never answered his phone. You wrote him to file your complaint but he never answered as well. You sent a text message, and still no reply.

So, what now? Your best shot failed.

How do you proceed?

The next step is to go back to the drawing board armed with the current experience that you have. Figure out your next options at this point. Use the unanswered letter and texts as evidence of your actions.

You may even want to take legal action at this time. Note what legal options are available to you. Determine the effects of that action against your landlord. Also determine the tenant's rights that are afforded to you by the law.

There are 2 possible things that will happen at the end of any problem-solving exercise. They include the following:

You will have eliminated the problem

You have built your self-confidence knowing how you have the capacity to formulate solutions that may potentially resolve issues.

CHAPTER 20:

Attracting Good Energy

Never expend your energy on worry; rather, use it to develop yourself and live a great life.

Positive energy can improve how we feel and communicate with the people around us. In our daily dealings with other people, we receive the kind of energy we send out. This energy is usually within our entire body, spirit and mind and, when it vibrates out, it's usually felt by others around us.

The way we feel about the people around us is a result of the kind of energy we carry around and the energy that we pick up on from them. We may feel free and cheerful being around some people and feel awkward and cold when we're around other people. Maintaining positive energy will improve our total well-being and help us to communicate more positively with people.

On the other hand, negative energy negatively affects our entire well-being due to the feelings of resentment, discord and unhappiness that accompany it. So, your ultimate goal should be to resist negative energy and embrace positive energy.

You can achieve this by increasing your energy level and surrounding yourself with positivity. Here are nine daily ways to help you boost your inner vibration and help you to feel the energy flow around you.

Pay Attention to the Energy You Release

If you're releasing lots of negative energy, there's no way you'll attract positive energy. How others feel when they are with you tells a lot about the kind of energy you discharge. Do people feel calm and happy or gloomy and sad when they're with you? Your answer to this will help you know if you have to work on boosting your energy or not.

Negative energy will always impact your relationships negatively, and your attitude towards others is a reflection of who you are. Ask yourself: What kind of impression do I make on people?

If you're the type that always reaches out to people and creates great relationships, you may be releasing positive energy. If you're the type that people avoid, you may be releasing negative energy. Therefore, you must focus on emitting positive energy.

Change the Way You Think

If you spend most of your time thinking about negativity, you'll become a pessimist in no time. But if you spend most of your time thinking about the positive aspects of your life, no matter how hard that can sometimes be, you'll easily attract good things. Always ensure that the positive thoughts guide you in all you do.

If you're battling a bad situation, resist the urge to slip into pessimism. Instead, tell yourself that it's only a phase, and it will soon pass. Always engage in positive affirmations, especially when things go wrong. When you receive bad news, try not to dwell on it or catastrophize. Replace negative thoughts with positive ones. Let the inspiration for your actions come from positive and realistic thoughts about yourself.

Discard Negative Influences

Quit surrounding yourself with negative people, things or places will take away your happiness and total well-being. Some people are toxic, and you should be far away from them. These are people that always try to discourage you from everything that you do and look for every means to bring you down constantly. If you're not observant enough, you may begin to pick up bad habits from these toxic places, people or things.

When you disengage yourself from these negative influences, you'll be able to design the kind of life you want for yourself. At times, disentangling from these influences may seem difficult because they're a part of your daily life. If this is the case, avoid them at all costs and prepare yourself mentally if you cannot avoid running into them.

Increase Your Circle

As you discard negative influences, increase your circle of positive influences. Surround yourself with people of like minds that can influence you positively and inspire you to be the best you can be. Ensure that you hold these relationships in high esteem and nurture them.

These people should be able to be honest and authentic with you, but it shouldn't be done to spite you or make you feel less sure of yourself. The positive energy that radiates from this group will help you live a happier life.

Be Kind and Compassionate

Some little acts of kindness can have a significant impact on the receiver and the giver. Being kind and compassionate towards others has been proven to attract lots of positivity and good relationships. So, the more you give and show compassion to others, the better your physical and mental well-being will be.

Being kind is also a great way to motivate the people around you and inspire them to be kind to others. Smiling to people around you, serving someone a cup of tea or doing anything that makes people around you happy sends loads of positive energy to you, and this boosts your inner happiness.

Be Grateful

Each day, if you dwell too much on negative thoughts, you'll find it hard to see the things you ought to be grateful for. Devote most of your quiet time to thinking about the little things in your life and be thankful for them. Doing this will help you let go of harmful and toxic emotions.

Think of the good things and people in your life and why you are grateful for them. Doing this for a few minutes every day will help you a great deal. If you can't think of any right now, you can begin by keeping a gratitude journal and jotting down a list of things that make you happy and feel contented. Being grateful will help you reflect on the bad times you've had and how you overcame them all.

Discover Your Inner Strength

Taking your focus away from all the negative thinking that may erode your confidence level and cause feelings of insecurity and self-doubt and shifting to positive thinking that boosts your self-esteem and confidence is essential to developing inner strength. Inner strength is what will make you resilient in the face of stressful situations and help boost your energy level so that you can handle whatever comes your way.

Align Your Current Self With Your Future Self

The things you spend your time and money on will determine how far you'll go in life. These choices you make today will shape your life tomorrow. Ask yourself: What do I desire most in the world? Work towards being the person that your future self will be proud of by building healthy relationships and a healthy lifestyle.

Develop a picture in your mind of who you would like to be in the future and start taking steps to make it a reality. Doing this will help you exert more control over your life, and the more positive actions you take, the more positive the reality you will create for your future self.

Act in Good Faith

There's a general belief in business that both parties act in good faith as they work together. We all benefit from treating one another fairly, but only a few people understand that this principle should be followed as we interact daily personally or professionally.

Endeavour to be nice to everyone you meet and treat them with respect, and in most cases, you'll receive the same gesture. Even if someone wrongs to you, avoid retaliation as it won't make you feel better. They may be having a bad day and react negatively to you for this reason. So, when you act nicely to everyone, even when they react harshly to you, you can be sure to attract positive energy, and this will help a lot.

CHAPTER 21:

Information Overload

T he brain isn't designed to process a complex of information at the same time. When your brain is thinking of several things at the same time to process, you brain gets stressed. When your brain becomes stressed, your functionality is reduced. Your productivity is almost reduced to zero. That is because your brain is confused about the information to really process.

What is Information Overload?

The term Information Overload simply means the abundance of supply of too much information. It's obvious that we live in the information age, where we have access to endless news, videos, and others. Technology and digital age have made it possible for information to be within the reach of our fingertips. Social media and the internet are widely regarded as the most influential factors in this regard. We are more exposed to information and consume information daily. There is over dependency on information. People are connecting to the internet to access one information or the other. There is more information now to absorb than they were, 10, 15, 20 years ago. The brain, which is the center of processing is expected to absorb and process all this information at once. How possible is that? The brain is configured only to handle as much as it could. It is limited to the amount of information it can store in its memory. Then, we have the mind that pays attention to about three to four at once. Anything beyond that is suicidal. You become unfocused, your thoughts become unclear and your decision-making process becomes slower and poorer. The complexity of the information makes the decision maker to face difficulties in determining the next best possible action to take.

If you want to get things done faster and be more creative with your positive thinking, you need to curtail the amount of information you are assimilating. You need to set limits to the amount of information that you are absorbing. By doing this, you are spending less time in getting tasks done.

Causes of Information Overload

Several causes of information overload abound. There are as many causes as there are the benefits. Being current with the latest news isn't a problem. The problem here is we are taking so much that our brains can't process. No one is able to take in as many as thousands of news every day. So why do we still stress our brains out even though it has reached its limit? Digging for information can be overwhelming and it leads to confusion and of course, information overload.

Causes of information overload includes;

Pressure to stay updated – You always want to be the first to know when something has happened. Factors like boredom is also responsible for this. You stay glued to news outlets and always want something to consume to satisfy your boredom. You are immersed in the flood of information because you are pressured to achieve one thing or the other. In the quest for knowing more, you are actually giving yourself information overload, which leaves you depressed, stressed, and confused most times.

Abundance of information channels that are available to us – Telephone, emails, social media networks are easily the most used channels for disseminating information. Email for example, receives more than 300 billion emails everyday worldwide. People constantly have problems going through their emails, keeping up with the rate of incoming emails, and filtering spam messages as well as deleting unwelcome messages. Workplaces, businesses, companies focus on the use of emails to reach billions of consumers, workers and business associates. Millions of people sign-up for newsletters on websites to receive latest news about a niche with the emails. The quantity of information one is exposed to through the channels makes it difficult for the person to think straight. Imagine filtering your email box for a whole day? It could have an impact on your thinking process.

The same thing goes for social media channel. Billions of information are passed through this channel daily and that's the reason behind information overload. You see different views on subject matters. Some that look confusing and some that look insulting. These things can cause information overload because you will be rooted in your thoughts, analyzing the information consumed, the different views, and reactions on the subject matter.

The Quest to disseminate and share information with friends and colleagues – You want to be in the circle of the "knows". You always want to be the first person to share an information with a friend, colleague or a relative and be tagged "the hub of information". The rapid growth of apps and dissemination channels such as Facebook and other social media networks has greatly influenced the quest to overshare information with other users. You want to be the first time always to hit the share button or the message button. The social media creates a distraction as people are consumed by the amount of information available to them, so much that they become the controllers of how they use such information. Social media overload has impacted productivity negatively and has resulted to poor decision-making process.

The desperation to accumulate more information for storage purposes – According to a famous game developer, people want to consume information, not because they need it at that moment, but because they need it, just in case something of sort springs up. Hence, they consume information for storage purposes. It's called, "the just in time situation versus just in case".

Most times, because the information you are consuming does not have an immediate purpose, you may find it hard digesting it and may even forget it on the long run. Take for instance, you learn a topic in school because it's mandatory and then, you learn another that is not mandatory or irrelevant to school setting. There is a higher chance of you retaining such information, because you know you would be needing it for a test or exams, compared to you learning a topic outside school because you feel you might need such information in the future. And because you are learning a topic that's outside a school setting and not related to what and why you need to learn at that moment, you will find it difficult learning.

The alarming rate at which new information is produced daily – The news media is a competitive industry, with companies trying to assert their authority. There is a premium put out on how fast news reaches the public. This leads to competitiveness among media houses in the news world. Media houses focuses on how to win the public with how reliable and fast the news reaches the public, so they would want to be on top of their "A" game. However, the quest for media houses to have a competitive advantage over the other, sometimes leads to the spreading of fake or false reports. The quality of the news is affected and we are left to deliberate if the report is actually true or false. At the end of the day, it's quantity over quality. During the process of analyzing information, we are overloading our brains with unnecessary thoughts. This is how information overload is caused.

How to Avoid Overloading the Brain with Information

There are a growing number of efforts and solutions globally to reduce information overload to the barest minimum. Some are suggestions and others are just trials. Some countries are putting some regulations to the use of Internet and the social media to curb information overload. However, the general solution to curbing information overload are;

Reducing the quantity of information absorbed

Only choose information that you need. Don't go about taking information because you want it. Rather, digest information because it's necessary. Rather than read up every story that trends online, pick out the one that's most important to you. That doesn't me you shouldn't how about seeking knowledge. The most important thing is you should not overload the brain with information that is not necessarily needed at the moment. Filter the quantity of information that you need. If it's impossible to filter news, shun the news media for just a day and you will see how effective you will become.

Employ a Cognitive Approach to Assimilating Information Better

Taking in information is not just the main thing. The main thing is how the brain processes the information. How does the memory retain the information that you just digested? This is where you need to employ cognitive methods to retain information in your brain.

Limit the amount of emails and sign-up newsletters

Despite the drop in the number of emails that is sent and received, a considerable amount of emails still overflows your inbox. The use of email has caused many to dedicate their time reading them and preparing replies. In order to curb this email addiction, limit the number of newsletter sign-ups and work on sorting out your mails. You shouldn't read every email that drops in your inbox. Sort out your emails according to importance in folders and delete any unnecessary email. Doing these comes with discipline. Which means that if you lack discipline, you won't have courage to sort out your emails. Disable any email notification, especially on your phone, because it's the number one source of distraction.

Reduce the frequent use of social media and disable Social Media Notifications

For individual profiles, it's necessary you prioritize updates from people you know and disable any notification. Notifications enables you to check what the notification is about quickly. Most times, you are stuck doing other things on social media like chatting with other friends online, reading news, watching viral videos, etc. Notifications are distractions and must be completely disabled or prioritized to effectiveness. The key here is to limit usage and the amount of information from friends shared.

Regulate the amount of time you spend on the Internet

The Internet is a very vast place with a lot of information from reliable and unreliable sources. Most times, the information you seek on the Internet is news. To reduce how much you rely on the Internet for news, choose a reliable news source and sign-up for their newsletters. This way, you are sure that the news you will be getting are not just false or unverified news. In the case of making an extensive research, use the Internet wisely and moderately.

Put Your Thoughts to Paper

Whatever that's going in that mind of yours, ensure you write it down. Those thoughts are interfering with your ability to focus. Then, set clear priorities. Determine if there are tasks that can be completed or not within a given time frame. Start from the smallest and ascend. Writing your thoughts down clears your mind and frees the mental space for other mental activities.

CHAPTER 22:

The Power of Goals

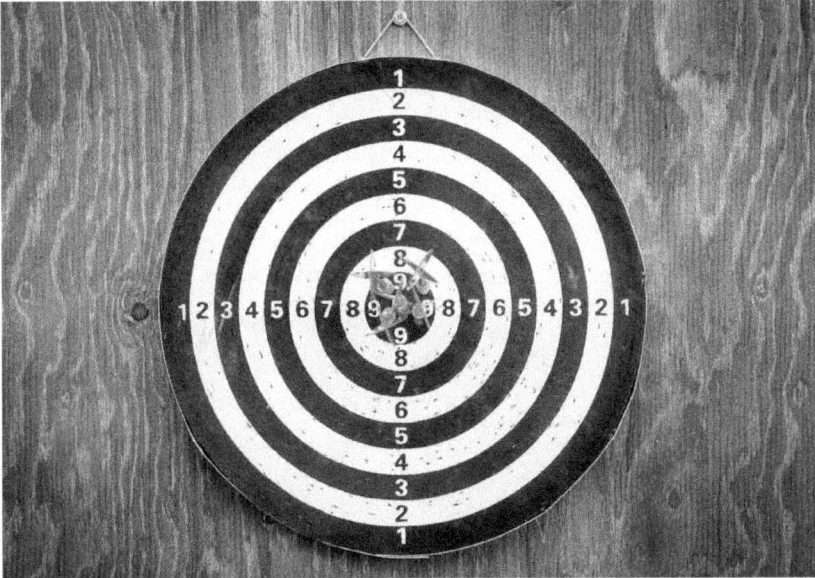

D o you really know how to set up your life goals? How frequently you can actually achieve the large-sized objectives which are actually important for you? When you face problems in setting up your goals properly, you might even get tempted to stop all your tries. In such situations, people have the tendency to say things such as, 'Maybe this is what it is' or 'I should be contented with what I already have.' In case your goal is to lose some weight, how will you understand that your goal has been completed? When you have lost 1 kg or 20 kg? When you fail to have a clear form of a target, you can never hit the right mark. That is why it is so tough to learn about the various things for setting up your goals which are measurable, clear and also actionable.

Why is it Necessary to have Goals?

An effective form of goal setting is the actual key to your success. Whether it is improving your intelligence, starting off with a new hobby, or restarting any relationship, when you set up goals, you can actually create the future right before it happens in actual. With goal setting, you can expand and grow in life which will be pushing you in the way which you might have never imagined before in your life. For the purpose of feeling fulfilled in the true sense, you are required to actually know what you are working on achieving something in your life. Progress in our lives is actually equal to happiness, and setting up goals besides it actually helps us in getting there. Most of the time, people think that they actually understand how to set up goals, but at the same time, they will not be achieving anything that they wanted. The very reason behind this is that the goals of such people were not inspiring or compelling nature.

Human beings are most likely to invest their energy along with time on something which actually excites them in real. So, all your goals need to reflect a similar level of excitement or momentum. You need to think of your goals as your dreams right with a definite deadline. All that you are required to do now is just to create up a blueprint for achievement.

Two primary questions for compelling nature of goal planning

Identifying the goals: What is the thing which you want to achieve? What is the objective which you actually desire? Looking out for a promotion at your work? Or to opt for meditation daily? For selecting the achievable form of goals, you are required to have a clear form of outcome in your mind. A very magical thing happens when you opt for something or when you take generalized nature of desires and then start to define the desires in a more precise way with the help of a detailed form of goal setting.

Identifying the purpose: Why are you looking out for achieving this goal? What is the result that you will receive after this? Will the promotion which you are looking up to give you freedom financially? For keeping your goals, you are required to ask the right form of questions, and then only you can seek real changes in life. When you know what you are actually moving towards, you will be able to find various ways in order to make the same thing happen. Always remember that the reasons always come in the first place, and they are the answers.

Goals and its Different Types

For further identifying how you can create the best process of goal-planning, you are required to know the actual type of goal which you want to achieve or have. There are various types of goals that can easily divide into several categories, like health goals, fitness goals, relationship goals, career goals, etc.

Short-term goals: This can be achieved typically within a period of less than one year, and it comes with things such as getting the promotion at work, lose 20 pounds, or building up a new home. While you look at the short-term goals in the process of goal planning, think of them as enabling your goals so that as you complete them, you can quickly move ahead for achieving the long-term goals.

Long-term goals: These are much more extensive in nature and generally take much more time to achieve when compared with short-term goals. Examples of this sort of goal would include starting your very own business, opting for a cruise for your wedding anniversary, and many others.

Lifetime goals: These goals are exactly of the type as they sound like. These are those goals that you actually want to achieve during the course of your life. It could be somewhat like retiring from your job at the age of 60 and then you want to participate in various mission trips with your partner. When it comes to the planning of goals for the lifetime goals, it would generally include the setting of capstone goals which are of similar nature as of enabling your goals.

How to Set the Right Goals

For the sole purpose of setting up the right form of goals, you need to follow certain steps:

Decide: First, you are required to think about something which you want to work on or want to achieve. It does not actually what you choose, unless and until you want to do it. It might be something which you are really interested in or actually feel excited about. But, make sure that it is within your limits or reach. The goals that you decide for you needs to be for its very own sake and not actually for something which others are doing. It might be small or big in size. It has been found that when you divide your goals into small pieces, it actually helps in achieving them as when you set up goals, which stretch can be motivating in nature.

Write them down: It has been proved that when you write down your goals instead of just thinking about them in your mind, there are high chances for you to stick to them. You need to write the benchmark for your goal, which will let you know when you have reached the destination and also the time when you will want to achieve the same. Write down how the goal actually connects with your life and describe them as much as you can. For instance, write down 'I want to plant some flowers in my garden in the month of May' instead of just writing 'I want to do gardening.' The more you write, the more it will be easier for you to achieve them. It will also allow you to plan up your goals and you can set up your schedules of life according to that.

Telling someone: When you share your thoughts with someone, it is most likely to make you feel motivated and positive. In the same way, try to share your goals with someone in your life who actually matters to you. When you tell someone about your goals, it will help in increasing your chances of sticking to the same. It also helps in bringing about a positive change in your life, which you need for achieving certain goals in your life. It will also help you in feeling more determined, and you will find it easier.

Breaking down your goals: This is a very important step for all the big type of goals. Try to aim on all the short-term or smaller goals, which will be necessary for achieving the bigger goals. The bigger sized goals might turn out to be a bit vague at times, such as, 'I want to be much healthier.' When you break down such goals into smaller goals, it will be easier for you to achieve the same. So, a smaller sized goal like 'jogging daily' will help you in your venture. Write down all the smaller goals and also assign time for each by which you want to achieve them. The faster you reach your smaller goals, the faster you will be attaining the bigger goals. Having small sized goals actually makes the whole journey a bit easier and will also give you a sense of success on the way.

Planning the first step: When you decide to walk 10,000 miles, you will need to put your first step. Even when your goal is not to achieve the 10,000 miles mark, just thinking about the very first step on your way can actually help in getting started with the journey. Even when you have no idea about where to start from, do not give any kind of excuse to yourself. You can do a research about the same before putting forward your first step. Always remember, when you try to give excuses to yourself, you are actually lying to yourself. Instead of just thinking about what to do, try to do something so that it can be regarded as your very first step. As you plan your first step, the rest of the journey will turn out to be easier for you.

Keep going: When you start working on your goals, it might turn out to be really frustrating and difficult at times. So, all that you are needed to do is to preserve. When you find out that a step of yours is not actually working, try to look out for something else which can actually help you in moving forward a little bit. In case you find yourself struggling with something on your journey, ask for help from people who actually have some idea about your goals. In case you find yourself to be really stuck with something on the journey, try to take a break. After you are done with your break, try again. Trying only can help you in achieving what you want in life. Even if you fail, do not stop and just keep moving. When you fail, your chances of winning also increases a lot than before.

CHAPTER 23:

Practicing Grit and Resilience

Thomas Edison failed 1000 times before he invented the light bulb. J K Rowling's Harry Potter was rejected 12 times before it was finally published. Henry Ford faced bankruptcy five times before he put Ford on the world map. When we look at these extraordinary people who have achieved greatness, we only see the result but not the journey. You may never know what it took someone to get where they are today because it is human nature to prioritize the result over the process.

We often assume that some people are so successful because they have outstanding brilliance or talent. Yet, the truth is that it is not the talent or the brilliance that makes them achieve greatness but rather their unwillingness to quit or surrender. Imagine the kind of mindset that it takes to be rejected twelve times and still try for the thirteenth. That is the secret behind people who achieve greatness. Their extraordinary resilience and perseverance in situations when anyone else would simply call it quits.

A lot of people are talented and many are skilled yet few make it to the very top. This is because true greatness comes at a price that few of us, no matter how talented are willing to pay; perseverance. Most people will never get to be rejected twelve times for the simple reason that they will never try that many times at anything. You may try twice or even thrice but for most people failing once is usually enough reason to give up. Perseverance is a skill very few people muster because it is not easy, or quick or convenient.

What makes these people that we celebrate everyday outstanding is not that they are more talented or more skilled than everyone else. It is their determination to succeed and the unwillingness to surrender that sets them apart from the average Joe or Jane.

Grit is about getting comfortable with failure and accepting it as a normal part of the process that leads to success. People who are willing to take extraordinary chances are those who are not daunted by the possibility of failure. They are not interested in playing it safe or sitting by the edge of the pool. They dive in again and again until they get what they want. This willingness and ability to keep trying time and time again is what defines mental strength.

When you have failed time and time again but you do not accept defeat as an option, then you have achieved mental toughness. Think for a minute, what do you do when you are rejected? When you are under pressure and running out of options how do you react? Do you fold and give up or do you get up and try again? Extraordinary things are only achieved through extraordinary resilience and perseverance. That is why there are only a few amongst us who will ever achieve greatness.

The No-Surrender Mindset

Actor Will Smith once asked how he manages to keep his marriage together in an industry where divorce is the norm. He answered that divorce was never an option for him and his wife. So, once it was off the table they had to work on their issues and come to a solution no matter what. In many ways, this explains the no-surrender mindset. What happens when giving up is not an option? Naturally, you focus on fixing the situation because that is the only option you have.

The thing about quitting is that if you do it often enough, it becomes a habit. The more you give up, the easier it gets to do the next time. That is why you will find some people try one thing after another without ever seeing anything through. Not because they do not have the talent or the skills required, but rather because they have made a habit out of quitting. When the going gets tough, the only option they see is quitting because they have trained themselves to shy away from adversity or difficulty.

Perseverance starts with passion and commitment. The goals you set for yourself should be so important that nothing can deter you from pursuing them. Your goals should be the things that you see in your mind the first thing when you wake up and the last thing when you go to sleep. They should be things that you are passionate about.

One common mistake that people make is setting goals that hold no true meaning for them. You want to do something because it is important to someone else, or because you feel you should but not because it is important to you. With this kind of goal, you will always find it difficult to persevere. You can only be committed and driven when what you are working towards is truly important to you.

Make yourself responsible for your life and your outcomes. Forget fate, or luck, or destiny. Whatever it is that you want out of life make it your business to make it happen. People with a no-surrender mindset understand that they must be in control of themselves in order to get what they want. They cannot wait for things to happen and react to them. They have to be proactive and keep the ball rolling.

Ultimately the no-surrender mindset is built on the principle of not giving up. Remove quitting from your list of options and start again. Not once, not twice, but as many times as it takes to get it done.

Disrupting Yourself

Insanity is often described as doing the same thing over and over and expecting different results. How is your belief system, attitude, and the image you have created for yourself working for you? Are you where you should be? Do you feel that you are on the right path? If you are unhappy, why are you accepting the situation instead of doing something about it?

Resilience is not just about being able to bounce back from failure but also being capable of reinventing yourself. Disrupting yourself means stripping away all the labels and attitudes you have covered yourself in and starting afresh. When your pen breaks, would you still keep trying to write with it? Of course not, because it is broken and not serving any purpose. So why are you holding on to beliefs, attitudes, and emotions that are not getting you anywhere?

For many people when they face difficulties, they always want to change the situation. You want to change jobs because your boss is a bully, or you want to change your major because what you are doing is too hard, or you want to change your diet because it is not working and you want to try another. In all these cases it probably never occurs to you to think about changing yourself instead of the situation. Why? Because it is always easier to try to change others than it is to change ourselves.

Resilience starts with an ability to see your weaknesses and the willingness to change in order to make yourself better. Examine your attitudes and the beliefs that make you who you are. Are you quick to generalize and make assumptions about people? Do you always have to win every argument to feel good about yourself? Do you know how to compromise? Can you say sorry when you are wrong? Are you still holding on to emotional baggage from your past relationships?

All these little things combine to influence how we see the world. They taint our experiences by making us only see what we want to see and overlook anything that goes against our beliefs. This is the kind of fixed mindset that makes people risk-averse. They are so used to thinking and acting in a certain way that doing something out of their norm is almost impossible.

Failure is only useful when you can use it as a lesson. Each time you fail, look for what you did wrong and what you did right. Carry the strengths forward and leave the weaknesses behind. Eventually, you will find that each time you fail you come out a little stronger because you identified something that stopped you from succeeding and you ditched it. If you cannot learn from failure and change who you think you are, you will always feel like you are banging your head against an invisible wall.

Stop Making Emotional Decisions

If you stop to examine all the times you have given up or quit, you can always trace it back to negative emotions. You were afraid to fail so you did not try, or you got angry when you were rejected so you gave up, or you felt miserable so you ended up binge eating and so on. Most of the emotional decisions that we make are driven by a need to make ourselves feel better in the moment.

When you make emotional decisions, you seek out instant gratification. You find it hard to persevere because you only want to experience the parts that feel good. This is the problem that many people face when trying to achieve a certain goal or stay on the right track. They simply cannot regulate their emotions.

Mental strength requires discipline because without discipline you will always be a prisoner to your emotions. It is discipline that will make you go to the gym even when you do not feel like it, or show up to work on time every day or study instead of going out partying.

Discipline is the only real weapon you have against your emotions and this makes it the foundation of mental toughness.

Develop a routine that sets out a clear path to follow. With time you will realize that mental strength is like a muscle. The more you use it the stronger it becomes. Overcoming your emotional impulses will be hard at fast but once the routines you have set in place become entrenched habits you will find yourself doing the right thing almost automatically.

When you rely on motivation or willpower you will only do things when they feel good or when you feel like it. However, if you establish clear routines and schedules, then you will have a deliberate path to follow that leads you from where you are now to where you want to be. Make it a mission not just to have goals but also to have a plan and a deliberate course of action.

CHAPTER 24:

What Makes You Bold and Fearless?

Boldness is not just about the action, but about the mindset. When you are bold and fearless, it means your mind is built to overcome doubts and insecurities. There are evident things you can do that make you feel and look bold. These actions will stimulate the best in you, and it will manifest as a habit, therefore ruling out all self-doubt and nervousness.

Self-love

Love yourself and all that you are. You are not perfect; nobody is perfect. Shift your focus from your flaws and align your concentration on the best you can do to make you happy. Do not criticize yourself. Do not harm your confidence by negative self-talk. Always think more of yourself, and people will think more of you.

When you respect yourself, you will treat yourself better; people will see the value you put upon yourself, and they will treat you with respect. You don't need people. You only need yourself to be at your best, and you will attract the right company.

Family comes. First, friends come second; stuff comes third

Put your family first. Love them and shower them with all the care you have. Protect their interests and never intentionally do anything that will hurt their feelings or goals. Your family should be your priority, then friends.

Give your friends the love you would give to yourself. Make a few close friends and treat others as acquaintances. You don't have to bring everyone close. Have as many connections with people as possible, for the speed of your success will be determined by the number of people you know and their qualities.

Materials possession comes last. Do not put too much value on perishable objects. For stuff comes and go, but only the wise hold on to better things.

It's okay to ask for help

Nobody is an island. Even the confident, brave and courageous ones ask for help. Everyone needs help in one way or the other. That is why the most successful people hire personal assistants to help them in running technical errands. With people's help, there is a guarantee for task facilitation.

You do not have to sweat anymore once family or friends are supporting you. You will be happier, feel loved, and create a deeper connection with these people. The brave and courageous do ask questions. It takes brevity for someone to be vulnerable to learn.

Do more

Do more to people who don't expect much from you. Meet the deadline and even do more. Give someone below you a chance to shine. Help someone in need, there is never a small help. All help lead to strong self-confidence and the feeling of value. Surprise your friend or loved ones once in a while.

Make someone's day by buying small gifts, to let them know you are thinking of them. Be passionate and let yourself go. Don't keep a record of the good things you have done. Be spontaneous about them, and do not expect anything in return.

Appreciate the smaller things

Appreciate the small achievements. Enjoy every single reward you get for working hard. Allow yourself to enjoy minor things like a good smell, a well-cooked vegetable, normal breeze, someone's smile, a glass of chill water, etc.

The best in life come out of the little things we enjoy. You will be happier about your life, and you will stay in proportion. Your level of anxiety will drastically drop because you are not concentrating on the problem anymore. Instead, you are concentrating on the good things, the beautiful, simple things.

Chase your dreams

One of the things that make life meaningful is our dreams. We have lots of dreams and fantasies. Set a realistic goal to achieve your dream. This means taking a simple step each day and enjoying your progress. Dreams don't have to be overwhelming. The journey towards your dreams should be exciting.

You will make mistakes, be prepared to learn from them. You will feel frustrated, remember the feeling; you will remember it when you finally make it. Listen to advice, commit to due diligence, and then apply the best. Prove yourself to yourself, and not to others. Prove that you can be great, that your thoughts can be transpired into reality.

Settle for learning

Since you are not perfect, you must make a mistake. The occurrence of mistake or error is an indication of admittance or missed step. You cannot benefit from a mistake by beating yourself about it or giving up. Errors come in handy once you take lessons from it. Take a step back and reflect on each step you took.

Write down some of the reasons you didn't succeed, then set a goal to try again. Your second performance will always be better. Develop a habit of repeating things until you get the accuracy you desire. That way you don't have to be afraid of making mistakes. You will thrive socially, and you will stop avoiding most of the things you avoid today.

Make happiness your choice

Happiness is a choice. If you think you deserve happiness, your endeavors will be predisposed towards the pursuit of satisfaction. Your motivation will shift from frivolous spending or seeking approval from strangers, to making yourself and the people closest to you happy.

If the people you love are happy, then who else do you need to make happy? No one. Once you force yourself to make someone happy, you will lose your joy. Help others, but only when it feels good within you. Do not displease yourself while trying to displease others. Choose the path to happiness, and you will find it.

Let love lead

Love is the greatest gift of humanity. People have annoyed you, and you are pissed right now, or maybe you've been angry with a family member for quite a long time. Now is the time to let love lead.

Anger impairs your judgment. Learn to accept people for who they are. Learn to accept yourself for the best you are. The situation is difficult, but do not let love depart from you. Forgive people, even yourself.

Be a helping hand

Ignore your issues for a moment, and assist somebody. One of the ways to improve confidence is dedicating your time to other people. The feeling of importance improves your self-esteem, and you will personally feel more responsible.

You will start making good choices since you know many people will depend on you. It is an ultimate sign of leadership, and you will begin to adapt other leadership skills to make yourself more dependable.

Improve your listening skills

Good listeners are the best conversationalists. They listen to people attentively and understand the meaning of their words and the meaning of their posture. They understand the gesture, and quickly develop empathy.

Good listeners don't argue much. They can disagree with someone, but they tend to listen more to the other side's point of view before commenting. Mostly, people agree with them, because they make points based on understanding how the other person is feeling and why the other person have certain qualities. When it is time to give advice, they never hesitate to hit the nail right on the head, but they are patient enough to wait for the right time.

Allow growth to happen

Growth is the process of improvement in all areas of life. Some people grow while others remain stagnant. Knowledge is the best vitamin in life. There are two types of people in this world, those who growth in 5 years, and those who repeat 1 year 5 times.

Are you in the same position you were today last year? What changed? Did you experience significant growth or improvement? Did you plan or work toward the growth? Where do you see yourself today next year? If you don't have a concrete plan to improve, you will be running around the same cycle

Learn to speak up

Speaking is not about knowing the facts. It is about sharing your feelings about other facts or opinions. Your opinion is gold. Speak up, and give yourself a chance to change the world. Do not underestimate your point of view. You might be the solution to the lingering problem in your workplace.

If you don't speak up, people will take advantage of you. Be assertive with your feelings, and forward in your action. If someone is trying to irritate you with their opinions, leave the room.

Be a finisher

Learn to finish everything you have started. A peaceful mind is a mind that finishes things, and have no lingering tasks. Fulfill your promises. Make sure you complete your to-do lists before the end of the day.

If you have a weekly to-do list, make sure everything is complete before the week runs out. Leaders are spotted through this lens. People would love to learn from you. So, you will be attracting enthusiastic people wanting to improve their lives in one way or the other.

Change what you don't like

Not everything is out of control. You can be shy and scared and still have control over some things in your life. If you don't want the way things are going, change them. Attain power over your personal life, and you will find it easy to make changes in your relationships and professional life.

Your freedom comes from the responsibility you take of your feelings. Your confidence will come from the conscious ability that you have control over everything.

If you like it, don't change it

If you like who you are, don't allow social influences to push you to change. No matter what you become, people will not be pleased. Be yourself, and the people who love you truly will love the person you are. The only challenge is to become the best of who you can be. Always expose yourself to activities that will bring about improvement.

You cannot change some imperfections or defects. Don't stress yourself trying to change what God intended to be permanent. Your natural defect makes you unique. You will be easily recognizable, and you will stand out in the crowd.

Don't be Afraid to Apologize

Apologize if you are wrong, even to a kid. Do not hold back your apologies, because brave people admit their mistakes. It shows that you are human and you can be vulnerable and remain strong.

One of the ways to get out of your comfort zone is apologizing. Although there will be a need for courage, you have to take the chance for the sake of improvement. Prove to yourself that you can be wrong and fearless at the same time.

CHAPTER 25:

Rewired to Win

Your Competitive Advantage is All in Your Mind

People in business-whether in leaderships, employees or entrepreneurs are motivated to prevail in various manners. In this, they share a great deal in common with those people who practice the martial arts. How about we inspect and look at these two fields and see precisely what they share in common and can empower you as a success-oriented achiever.

How are the best business professionals and martial artists alike?

Both practice mental conditioning, consolidating those abilities with their experience and knowledge to successfully reach their objectives. If you are training others, the strengths of martial arts will fabricate their abilities. If you as of now have an effective business, understanding the standards of martial arts and bringing them to bear on your day by day errands could drastically expand your influence and success.

Some of the advantages that business experts gain from martial arts are like the characteristics that individuals associated with both the best martial artists and the best business experts: a ground-breaking presence; an ability to manage emotions under tension; the courage to handle tough situations judiciously, and the ability to adjust to evolving circumstances. When practiced every day, the two disciplines: Build resiliency to be able to bounce back from difficulties rapidly; Enable you to turn into an agent of change and to coordinate change; Refocus your thinking as the circumstance changes; Channel your attention to manage the circumstance.

Martial Arts as a Science and an Art

Martial Arts - Karate, kick-boxing, taekwondo, and so on - is both a science and an art. Utilizing it as a science, martial artists train to build up their techniques in figuring out how to situate their hands, feet, and body to perform a punch, execute a turning kick, or dodge a punch or kick without losing their balance. Martial artistic practice the various procedures until the feeling of the method and its execution become hard-wired. Utilizing it as an art, they practice much like a dancer, painter, sculptor, or musician-refining their art with everyday best practices to reinforce their muscles, reflexes, and abilities constantly.

It's the equivalent to business experts. The effective ones constantly strengthen their muscles, reflexes, and abilities in the everyday operations of their business. Strong business experts apply their abilities dependent on in-depth studies and research. These incorporate such regions as engaging worker motivation, executing change management, being a pioneer who encapsulates and promotes transformational initiative, running viable meetings, and conveying superb client assistance.

This implies in the art of martial arts and business experts, it takes preparation, training, applying, and coaching what is learned. Through practice, military artists hard-wire their strategies in their brain by persistently sharpening their aptitudes; and while genuine business expertise originates from something other than just reading books or taking an interest in a telecast, business experts hard-wire in their brains what they realize by constantly applying the knowledge so they can act with more confidence, precision, and influence.

Your competitive benefits start first in your mind

In the book Hard Optimism, Price Pritchett writes,

"The brain is currently the main productivity tool. Thinking has become the key competency. Individuals' thinking processes are the most significant performance factor."

This implies all human action starts in the brain - an intersection of our ideal results, creative mind, and imagination. Martial artists visualize the desired result and practice successful strategies thousands of times to solidify the wiring between the brain and the body with the goal that it gets programmed. Although various martial arts rules collectively transfer to life and the business world, there are three key standards or mental aptitudes that underlying affect business experts and throughout everyday life.

- Awareness
- Mental Toughness
- Focus

Business school, as well as your business experience, showed you these psychological abilities, to a certain extent; the business experts who learn them well and practice them consistently succeed. Whether your fundamental work is driving your business and team – planning, researching, setting goals, and strategizing - or participating actually as a sales rep or active producer - you can utilize these three mental standards to upgrade your performance.

To become a winner in business and life, you should initially become a champ in your brain. However, to change your reasoning, you should first re-wire your brain.

Re-Wiring your Brain to Create New Pathways

Brain specialist Dr. Jill Ammon-Wesler, in her book, Zap Your Life: Feel the Power! composes that,

"Your brain normally blossoms with change and challenge. Current science presently has evidenced our brains always develop and change well into old age. The brain is very variable that the logical world needed to make another term - "brain plasticity"....our brains constantly re-wire themselves within hours following each new experience."

What it really implies to you is that you can re-make yourself, make a new path, and show your desires right there in your brain! Imagine: What might it be want to re-wire your brain into the psychological focal point of an Olympic athlete, or to experience business clarity like Bill Gates?

Neurologically, our brains have just been molded by past patterns of thought, attitudes, mood, and emotions. In the womb, our genetic DNA starts assembling our brain and developing certain neurological pathways. After birth, every one of us gets sensory information and various encounters that keep on building our brains. Our responses and reactions to those encounters further build our brains. The soonest, most grounded and most repetitive encounters - and our reactions - hard-wire our brain.

An illustration is when little children, who experience issues in understanding cognizance and whose imperfections are persistently called attention to by authority figures, in the long run, develop "profound trenches" of poor self-image and self-esteem - reflected in negative self-talk - which become a significant part of their brain's composition. While they can fabricate new roads through positive reasoning - and set down new pathways and propensities to challenge, diminish and even defeat negative ones - the old ruts are never erased.

Neurological pathways remain, and even new encounters can fall into those old negative ruts of reasoning.

This is a significant idea in understanding how our mind works. One of the general laws of the mind is this: Whatever your mind constantly contemplates will often become reality. If for instance, you always feel that your item won't sell, it won't. You have made a psychological desire - your reasoning turns out to be initial a rut and afterward a self-fulfilling prophecy.

To rewire your brain and to change this negative result, you should stop the negative idea and train yourself to think differently. What result do you need from them? When you depict the result you need, your perspectives won't just incline toward accomplishing it, but your brain will start thinking through the best possible steps to make the goal a reality.

Imagine a Wall Street ticker tape. Substitute the stock images on the ticker tape for individual contemplations. Similarly, an interminable loop of positive and negative thought circles in our minds. In all actuality, every one of us can intentionally, deliberately apply exertion to change our thoughts, sort out them into sound patterns, and afterward control how we process those thoughts at any moment. In the martial arts we are trained not exclusively to control the nature of our reasoning, but in addition to deal with our feelings. This originates from the act of being constantly aware of what we think and how we feel.

For instance, Carla is a new leader at a media transmission organization who is asked by her supervisor to present at an organization meeting. She has presented before to a smaller audience, but this is her first experience with a huge crowd. She feels the weight of needing to perform well. Instead of harping on dread and jumbling her mind with what if she returns to a beginner's mind. She prepares herself up in her imagination she re-encounters her moments of pinnacle execution when she exhibited effectively. As she feels the vitality at this moment, she envisions applying them in her new presentations. She realized she needed to connect with her past habits to assist her with growing new ones. She realized that if she distinctively envisioned having another habit, her brain would normally start to rewire to make the physical and mental connection.

John is a business proficient for a manufacturing production network organization that is profoundly partitioned on a significant choice, feeling conflicted and uncertain of his methodology. He knows that his considerations are unfocused and running in various ways while the negative voice inside his head is yelling doubt and fear. He stops it, clears his psyche with a beginner's brain, and sets up useful information-gathering questions that lead to successful improved performance and decision making. Everything that both of these people did was a result of their psychological habits. Despite your field of intrigue, the martial techniques gives important lessons to anybody confronting difficulties from business, sports, to the fields of art and politics.

The Weak or Undisciplined Mind

An undisciplined or frail mind is like an "interior foe" or an "internal voice" that authorizes us or entices us to do less. Here are a few instances of a business expert's negative reasoning (your "inward foe"):

When you are tired, this "interior adversary" persuades you that two hours of preparation is sufficient, when you know that four is required.

You make an excuse for your behavior by utilizing your emotions or outside conditions as motivation to be less productive.

You complain about the number of hours you are spending on a presentation or contract.

You plan to test for the bar exam in 2 months, but you have neglected to focus on an extraordinary daily study plan.

Rewire your brain by subbing each negative idea with a genuinely charged positive one - and quickly follow up on the positive idea. In the end, with less exertion, your positive idea will turn out to be hard-wired, and you will at that point start to act in an amazing, concentrated way - the consequence of an incredible, centered personality.

Focus and Effective Thinking

Foolish reasoning is characterized as having uncontrolled, unfocused contemplations. This sort of reasoning happens when you come up short on an unmistakably characterized objective or have not considered all the particular steps you should take to achieve that objective. You are thinking foolishly when you are occupied with a discussion and can't distill its main points, when you delegate undertakings to others without having adequately considered the assignments, or when you make a half-hearted commitment.

Effective reasoning envisions procedures and steps. You have prepared and planned to pose the correct inquiries pertinent to a testimony or conference. You can brainstorm successfully because you realize what the ultimate objective is. When you delegate, you have considered not just what you need a partner to achieve, but how you will monitor that undertaking and give useful input along the way. When you practice these three disciplines habitually, your competitive advantage is "All in your brain." And you're certain to be re-wired to win.

CHAPTER 26:

Troubleshooting

Get Back on Track

L et's say you did everything, you practiced the techniques in this book, and then out of nowhere everything seems to be falling apart. Your negative thought-patterns came back, you have started to worry and overthink everything again, and you just need a quick pick me up - Here is how to get back on track in three easy steps:

1. Identify the problem, and find the root cause

Usually, when we try to do something new, our old habits try to sneak their ways back into our lives, making it that much more difficult to continue changing our habits. This is because we haven't found the root of our problem. Try to re-identify the root of the problem by addressing your triggers. Here are some trigger examples that may be causing you to fall off track:

- Stress from changes and relationships;
- Boredom from lack of progress;
- Chronic illness or injury;
- Change in environment, like moving or vacationing;
- Doing too much too soon.

To avoid your old habits creeping up on you, take some "me time" to figure out what triggered you to fail in the first place. Don't look at this as failure, but as a chance to start again with more knowledge.

2. Restart the behavior by practicing your positive-habit training

Go back to the basics and remind yourself that overthinking is not going to do anything but make you counterproductive. Don't ignore your thoughts, instead acknowledge them and practice mindfulness that they are there. Set a worry schedule and write your worries down to deal with during this time of worry. Practice meditation, and if you have been lacking, then dedicate yourself to some exercise. By doing these things slowly, it will force your brain to remember the habits you were trying to form and get you back on track to challenging your thought-patterns. When you have this down pat again, go back and make small goals and reward yourself when you accomplish them.

3. Try a different approach

Not all methods of action work for everyone, so find a different approach that suits you better. For example, if your worry time is right after dinner, around 6pm, start your worry time before dinner, around 3pm. Or maybe you woke up, started working out, then showered after that, but you fail because you find you're rushing your day due to this routine. So, work out just before you wind down for sleep. By finding a different approach, you may just find something that works best with your schedule, then getting on track will come easily.

Calm Anxiety (Worrying) in Five Minutes or Less

Anxiety and other mood disorders are common for enabling your old habits to return to the surface. This is because our anxieties allow us to do what is familiar and "safe." Anxiety doesn't like change and it will seem as though you are constantly having to restart because you give into your anxieties and fall back rather than shoot forward. The trick to overcoming this is figuring out ways to calm down immediately. Here are ways to do just that:

1. Play the 5-5-5 game

The 5-5-5 game is a grounding technique. Look around the room and name five things you can see. Close your eyes, take in a deep breath and name five things you can hear. Keep your eyes closed, or re-open them, move five body parts, and name them. (For example, move your wrists and say aloud "wrist," move your toes and say aloud "toes.") Start again and do this as many times as you can until you feel calm. Be completely in the present as if you are seeing, hearing, and moving for the first time.

2. Do a quick exercise

Jump up and down, spin in circles, stretch, pace, move the muscles in your face, wiggle every part of your body, dance, or any activity to get your body moving.

Do anything you can do for exercise, maybe go for a light jog or a brisk walk to change your surroundings.

Sometimes all your body needs is a little exercise to get past the initial adrenaline rush of anxiety. While you are exercising, pay attention to the weak feeling in your legs or the tingle in your fingertips. Move past this, and this trains your brain to overcome these uncomfortable feelings healthily.

3. Throw a cold cloth on your neck

By putting a cold cloth on your neck, holding an ice cube, or taking a cold shower, you are shocking the anxiety out of your system. Sometimes all your body needs is a quick shock to bring your attention away from the anxiety or worried thoughts.

4. Eat a lemon or a banana

Taste buds are a quick way to shock your system too. Eating a lemon will make your face scrunch and your body jolt, and so the worries or overthinking which are causing the anxiety will instantly stop. Bananas hold a ton of nutrients that will bring your sugar levels back to normal as well. Sometimes you may just be having a sugar attack from high or low sugar intake, so a banana will bring these levels back to normal, which will make you feel calmer.

5. Question your anxiety

Take a minute before you panic to address your thoughts. Question them. What is causing the anxiety? Which of the cognitive distortions do these thoughts fall under? Are you underestimating your ability to handle this right now? Is this a false alarm? What can you do about it? What is the worst that can happen? When you stop to answer these questions in full, you will notice that your mind doesn't have the attention span to send negative symptoms to your body and think about how to answer these questions at the same time. This may make you feel calmer. When these questions are answered, take a minute to focus on your breathing, sit down, and be mindful of your breaths.

Quick Methods to Decrease Negative Thinking

On those days where your thought-patterns have drowned out all the positive, and you find yourself falling into the mindless chatter surrounded by negative thinking, follow these easy methods to get out of it quickly:

1. Cut it off

This technique requires you to act quickly. The second you realize you are thinking negative thoughts, cut them off. Yell "STOP" inside your mind, or even out loud. Don't pay attention to the negative thinking, don't argue, defend yourself, or analyze it. Just cut it off as if it doesn't exist. Immediately think about something else or get up and do something else. Find a distraction so that you are no longer listening to your negative thoughts.

2. Label the thoughts

If cutting them off doesn't work, then try labelling them. Acknowledge that what you are thinking is negative, remind yourself that it is only a thought. You can choose to pay attention to it or ignore it, either way you don't have to act on it as it is only a thought and it does not define your actions. Negative thoughts only have power over you if you give them the control to dictate your actions. It isn't about how we challenge our thoughts, but how we react to them. When we do nothing about them, we gain our control back. So repeat to yourself, "This is only a negative thought, and I don't have to do anything about it."

3. Exaggerate the thoughts

Another way to take control of your negative thinking is to exaggerate the original thought simply. For example, imagine you are trying to learn something, and you just don't get it. You have been at it for hours and you notice yourself thinking, "There is no point in trying, I am just stupid and will never learn." Acknowledge that this is negative, and then exaggerate it outrageously and make it humorous. So say, "Yes; in fact, I am so stupid that I couldn't even screw in a light bulb if I tried. And because I am this dumb, everyone will notice so that they will laugh at me. After they are finished laughing, I will give them a reason to laugh and start hopping around like a kangaroo, yelling like a donkey, to the point where everyone, including myself, will laugh. Then after that, I will show myself just how silly stupid I can be." Continue like this, using your imagination and being as sarcastic as you can, not taking anything, you purposely say personal. When you do this, I bet you your mind will be quiet after this.

4. Counteract

This technique is the opposite of the last technique. When your mind says, "I am so stupid," say the exact opposite and nothing more. So that would look like, "I am the smartest person in this room." If your mind says, "I will never be good enough," then say, "I will always be good enough." When your mind says, "I'm too stupid to understand this stuff," say, "I am too smart to understand this stuff." This works because when we think too much about our negative thoughts, we usually fear ourselves acting them out. And when we fear acting upon them, the fear usually comes true because we end up doing what we try so hard not to do because we give it too much attention. So when we say the opposite to our thoughts, we aren't really paying attention to them, rather we are forcing our minds to think positively.

5. Enforce positive affirmations

For every negative thought, come up with two positive affirmations. So when your mind says, "I am not good enough," say, " I am grateful to be enough for the world today," and, "It's a good thing I am beautiful, because this negative thought could really get the best of me if I let it." The reason we come up with two positive affirmations for every one negative thought is to be more focused on positive thinking than negative thinking. Over the course of your day, you may feel so good about yourself that you give yourself credit for making yourself feel this way.

Conclusion

We have now come to the end of this book, but this is only the beginning. You may not find yourself taking different actions, or changing anything tangible in your life, externally, at first, but if you apply this and practice it, you're going to feel better. You're going to notice where you have the tendency to focus more on the negative side of things than the positive side of things. And you can change that.

You've been in the driver's seat all along. Now you know it.

It's significant to understand that there's likely some momentum in-place. You've been thinking and feeling and thinking and feeling in habitual ways perhaps for a while now, which has created a certain flow of energy.

But here's the great thing: it stops when you think other thoughts. Easy as that.

If you put just a little less attention on the things that feel bad, and a little more attention on the things that feel good or better, the momentum of the unwanted naturally becomes less.

Picture two fire pits, equally burning. The one on the left is your "negative" thoughts and feelings, and the one on the right is your desired thoughts and feelings (the ones that feel better to you). Once you decide you want to feel better, you've taken a step toward adding fewer sticks to the left-side fire pit. If you add only the occasional stick to the fire pit on the left and intentionally add more sticks to the fire pit on the right, eventually, the one on the left is going to go out, and the one on the right is going to burn better.

It's not that you're getting rid of the fire on the left by doing something. It's just going to stop burning because of your lack of attention and tending to it. In giving less attention to the one, you're giving more attention to the other. It's that easy.

It can take time, and it doesn't always feel easy, because of that momentum, but if you substitute something you've been thinking or doing, with something else, soon what-was won't be, because you've replaced it with something else. It's about replacing an old habit by forming a new one.

You'll still do things, think, perceive and feel things out of habit — like how you habitually turn on the light switch, even when you know your power's out — but eventually, you'll stop because your new habits will have replaced your old ones.

That's why you need to be steady when it comes to this work. Mastery isn't about perfection, it's about understanding that mastery is never done.

It takes consistency. It takes the intention to step on the stone to cross the stream, and then move to the next stone, or if you can't move to the next stone, hang out for a while, with the intention to keep heading across at some point. If you keep going back to the other side though, or if you try to jump too far, you'll face-plant and you'll believe "this shit" doesn't work for you. Or that you're not good at it. When, in fact, it IS working perfectly and you can get "good at it." You can go to the "bad-feeling" side of the stream, and things will play out in your life that match how you feel. You're still demonstrating your power either way. It's just whether you want to feel better or worse.

You have to care enough about how you feel and want to feel good to think the thought that feels better, or change the subject to one that does. Consider this your new approach to being, not just something you do every now and again. Think of this as a lifestyle change vs. a fad that will eventually fade.

Things are going to happen and trigger you, and you're going to feel bad. Embrace all your emotions, because they're all good. They're all helpful information. They're all feedback to empower yourself.

Things are going to happen that you might not have seen coming (wanted or not), as if they "came out of the blue." You know differently now.

Your capacity to feel good is limitless. And so is your capacity to feel bad. Which way you go is up to you.

This is just the beginning.

The key to living a good life is feeling good.

A happy life is nothing but a series of choices to feel good.

Everything you want is for that purpose. If you start making the correlation between your thoughts and how you feel, and how that affects your life, and if you have the desire to feel the best that you can, your life will progressively and endlessly continue to become what you want it to be.

The key is feeling good along the way. Not "when." Not "if." Not "as long as." Just because.

This truly is just the beginning. You can apply this knowledge to any part of your life, any subject, anytime, anywhere, no matter what. You are now aware that you're in control, you are now aware of your power to create, and you have the tools to apply it, and to let it be easy.

So enjoy this process. If you discover something here that works for you, live it, be it.

If others around you notice and want to learn where your mojo is coming from, then you can tell them. But unless they're asking, it's often better to keep it to yourself. Otherwise, you're going to be that jerk know-it-all who's discovered the secret to the universe and has to tell everybody. Let people discover it in their own time, at their own pace. Just live it in the best way you possibly can, for yourself.

Now go. Live your life.

Get what you want.

Create what you desire.

Know you're worthy.

And enjoy the ride. Because that's what it's always all about.

I'm excited for what you're in the process of discovering!

CPSIA information can be obtained
at www.ICGtesting.com
Printed in the USA
BVHW041014150321
602551BV00006B/497

9 781801 093590